Extreme Rapid Weight Loss Hypnosis for Women:

Feminine Affirmations for Weight Loss, Deep Sleep, Meditation and Motivation. Self-Hypnotic Gastric Band. Quit Sugar & Rapidly Burn Fat.

EASYTUBE ZEN STUDIO

Table of Contents

DISCLAIMER

I have undergone and tried all hypnosis techniques, meditations, affirmations, massage, yoga exercises, and other ideas presented in this book. I can attest that all strategies included in this book worked for me and others I know. However, I have no control over how these techniques affect some people.

This book is not claiming any financial gain or guarantees. It is also not intended to provide medical advice, treatment, or diagnosis. If you have a medical condition, consult with a health professional first before doing the strategies discussed in this book. We are not responsible for any misuse of information found in this book, especially for those who skipped going to the doctor despite their health risks.

> *Affirmation without discipline is the beginning of delusion.*
> *- Jim Rohn*

Weight loss is simple. Yes, you've read it right. If you have tried many times before to lose weight but failed is because you've been doing it wrong. It's not just about diet and exercise.

You are only dealing with the obvious problem when you resort to meal replacements, slimming pills, counting calories, out-of-this-world diet plans, and starvation. And that is your physical appearance.

You're overweight and fat.

When you recognize the problem and quickly think that your physical appearance is the problem, the first thing you will do is to restrain yourself from eating. You may also be inclined to try products that claim they can help you lose weight.

I was once like this when I was a teenager and didn't know any better. I was fat, and my high school bullies wouldn't skip a day reminding me of the obvious. The bullying got so bad that I simply stopped eating one day. And then I became sickly, and the bullies were onto me again. I was the fat kid who stopped eating.

It made me realize that other people would always have something to say whatever I do. Also, haters are going to hate, even if I become the fittest person in school. Why? Because they think highly of themselves. They say things without considering what the bullied would feel. I was hurt not because I was told I was fat. I already knew that. The bullying affected me because it hurt me inside. My confidence was already thin at that point, but their hurtful words made it fade. I allowed them to hurt me to the point that I stopped caring about myself.

When I stopped eating, I wasn't happy. My family wasn't happy. The only people who laughed at my misery were my bullies. Why? Because they hit me where they were aiming to hurt me - inside.

That was how I understood the problem was not because I was fat. It was more than that. I was hurting inside. And then I knew that if I didn't understand why I became overweight in the first place, I wouldn't get fit no matter how hard I tried.

When the problem is inside you, but you keep doing quick fixes to solve your physical dilemma, you are not solving the real issue. You have to know why you became fat in the first place. Only then will you be able to efficiently address the external problems, which is your physical form.

If you are not going to the roots of the problem, you will keep stumbling down even when you have decided not to eat at all. Me, I starved myself and lost some weight after several days. But then I became depressed, so I reached out for food and binged. I'd get guilty, so I'd starve myself again, but then I'd feel depressed and eat.

It became a cycle that keeps on repeating. And it did not solve anything. I became sickly. I did not get fit. I was still being bullied. The problem only worsened because I sunk into depression, and my confidence level reached far too low.

THE LIGHTBULB MOMENT

After understanding that I was fat because I was emotionally unstable, I made a goal. I promised myself to understand the issues why I overeat and resolve each of them. I also understood that I had an unhealthy relationship with food as much as I loved it. This means that I had no control. I'd eat whenever I wanted and did not stop even after feeling full. And my first response to my emotional troubles was to eat.

This book will teach you how you can regain your life and be in control. You will understand why you tend to overeat and try to overcome them one step at a time. This will teach you how to love food but not in an abusive manner. You will change your relationship with food in a way that will benefit you both inside and out.

It's not impossible to love eating out, enjoy cooking, or socialize around food and stay slim. I have seen a lot of slim people who are like that. They express their passion for food instead of suppressing it. They don't deny themselves, but they don't overindulge either.

Overeating all the time is a disability. You will only lose weight if you learn how to overcome it. This is what this book will teach you. It will change how your mind thinks about food and overeating. Once you've successfully dealt with the "demons" inside, you will develop a healthier relationship with food, gradually become fitter, and enjoy the benefits for a long time.

Before delving further into hypnosis and other ways to combat the roots of the problem, let's begin with affirmations.

THE IMPORTANCE OF AFFIRMATIONS

If you haven't tried doing affirmations, either in spoken or written forms, it's best to start soon and do it every day. Affirmations are inspirational statements we say or write that can change how we feel and view the world. They are healing.

An affirmation can be a sentence or any thought that makes sense. It is comprised of powerful words combined to form a positive statement. Affirmation works by motivating you by tapping into your conscious and subconscious mind. It pushes you to work harder, to get up when things seem heavy. It challenges and encourages you.

All of us have unhealthy and negative thoughts about ourselves. It's normal to be our number one critique at times. It only becomes a problem when we let ourselves get dragged down by these negative thoughts. You did not pursue a job application because your inner voice said you are not qualified. You stopped courting a person you liked because your inner voice said you weren't her type. You quit your fitness journey after hearing your inner voice telling you that it is too difficult and you won't make it.

While you can write down your affirmations, it will be more effective if you will say them out loud or chant them. You have to hear these affirmations, even when your own voice speaks them. The louder you say them, the more silent your inner voice will get. And that is the goal - to silence the inner voice that feeds you negativity and pessimism.

Once you attain the goal, the affirmations work by changing the way to think and act. You become more positive. You change all the negative behaviors and think and act positively. If you do this every day and chant your affirmations to remind yourself that you are good and you are destined for better and bigger things, it will be easier for you to dream and achieve greatness.

Affirmations have already helped a lot of people. They have endless benefits, the most important of which is that they allow you to continue making positive changes in life. They boost your confidence and help you become a better person.

THE SCIENCE BEHIND THE POWER OF AFFIRMATIONS

For many years, scientists believed that the brain was locked and unchanging. But we have surpassed the belief. Thinking can affect the brain's functions, as well as its structure and physical shape. According to neuroscience, doing an action requires the same sensory and motor programs in your brain as imagining it.

For example, when you close your eyes to imagine an apple, your brain's primary visual cortex will light up as it does when you are looking at a real apple in front of you. Here's another example. Writing your signature on a paper and imagining that you are doing the action using your dominant hand will take almost a similar time. This is the same when you do the action and imagine using your non-dominant hand. Both processes will take an almost equal amount of time.

What does this mean? Action and imagination are related and use the same neural pathways. Doing one action influences the other. One study used imagination to find out if it effectively strengthens muscles. Two groups were studied and given the same figure muscle exercises they had to do for a month. One group did the physical exercise, and one group only imagined doing the exercise. The group that did the physical training increased muscle strength by 30 percent. On the other hand, those who only imagined doing the exercises increased their muscle strength by 22 percent.

How is this possible? There are neurons in the brain responsible for the instruction of movements. In both groups, these neurons are used and strengthened, resulting in the strengthening of muscles despite one group not performing the exercises physically.

This is not something magical or mystical. It's science. It connotes that mental practice effectively prepares you for a physical task. Each thought changes your brain's function and structure by affecting the neurons at the microscopic level.

It doesn't mean that you can be the next musical genius after learning and practicing the piano in your mind alone. Those who review using their minds are already skilled musicians who are only trying to remember what they have learned after a lot of hard physical work.

USE YOUR MIND TO IMBIBE POSITIVITY

Let us begin your weight loss journey by learning various affirmations you can chant each day, depending on what you are trying to address. The affirmations will help you desensitize and surrender yourself from the bodily symptoms of whatever emotions you are trying to deal with. With continued practice of the affirmations, you will find your emotional attachment to your sensations of whatever you are going through. The attachment will be lifted once you have gotten rid of the emotional charge behind the feeling.

The process of removing the emotional charge is called desensitization. It will help turn your focus to more on your external world than your internal world.

It is best to chant or listen daily to the affirmations for 21 days. No matter how you do it, ensure you're comfortable while lying down or sitting.

Here are some affirmations you can say aloud or chant to deal with your anxiety, success, depression, and sexual issues or insecurities:

Whatever affirmations you're doing, close your eyes and be comfortable. Rest your analytical mind for a while as you listen or chant the affirmations. Let go of your worries and breathe deeply. At each breath, you become more and more relaxed as you let go of the thoughts in your mind and the feelings in your body. Surrender all your expectations and pre-judgments as you surrender to the words and allow them to go deep into your subconscious mind.

Anxiety Affirmations

I am safe.

I only allow myself to entertain positive thoughts.

I am an observer of everything my body feels.

I love myself unconditionally.

I become aware of my bodily sensations easily.

Everything I feel is normal, and I fully accept them.

I am letting go of my bodily feelings.

I float with my bodily feelings effortlessly.

It's okay to observe whatever feelings arise.

I have recognized most of my fears are mere illusions.

I now say goodbye to my fears.

My thoughts are now perfectly aligned for freedom.

With each breath I take, my body becomes more emotionally balanced.

I now find it easier to observe than to react to my body's feelings.

I am safe because it is alright to let go of the emotions I'm holding on to.

It's now easier for me to listen to my higher self.

I've got the greatest healing mechanism in my body that allows me to listen to my higher self.

I no longer need to seek someone's reassurance, for I know I am safe.

I surrender to my bodily feelings from this day on.

Starting today, healing happens naturally.

These affirmations show me the truth that I am safe.

It's now easy for me to focus my mind on things that matter.

I can now easily disregard the fearful voice that comes from within.

I now put all my focus on the voice of love and true understanding.

I know I am in good hands because I have learned to love myself more.

Feeling is natural, so I no longer make the mistake of thinking that it's not.

My bodily feelings are part of my life, and that's okay.

I am becoming more self-worthy with each affirmation.

I embrace change from now on.

Healing becomes easy when I am in this state.

I will become an inspiration for others from this day on.

I completely move to each feeling without questioning it.

The more that I love myself, the more understanding I become.

I am not a label.

I am limitless.

I am strong.

The world awaits for me to share my unique gifts.

Life becomes easier to live from this day on.

As I continue breathing, I become more confident that I can deal with anything.

I no longer feel the need to act differently to please everyone else.

I am now comfortable with all the bodily feelings I experience.

I am confident that I'll rise up to all the inner challenges I experience from now on.

I now put my faith in the intuition of my higher self.

Life is one exciting journey, and I now embrace its love for me.

My life is mine to live, and I will live it from this day forward.

I will no longer fall victim to any feeling in my body.

Open your eyes, and practice your new self to everyone you meet and everything you do.

Success Affirmations

Chant or listen to the following "I am" success affirmations at the start of each day for 21 days. The practice will allow you to ingrain powerful statements. Through the days, the affirmations will help you build results, confidence, and prosperity.

I am competent.

I am successful.

I am capable.

I am smart.

I see all opportunities and pursue them.

I am worthy of everything good happening in my life.

I am skilled.

I create worthy win-win relationships.

I am powerful.

I am strong.

I am worthy to succeed.

I carry the aura of being successful.

I deserve to succeed.

I confidently pursue what I want in life.

I set ambitious goals I am confident I can achieve.

I believe in myself.

I am accomplished.

I defy all challenges.

It is my nature to succeed.

It is my birthright to succeed.

Success prompts me to take action.

Success makes it easier for me to live life to the fullest.

Success makes it possible for me to make a positive impact in the world.

Feeling successful is who I am.

I am empowered to create all the prosperity I desire.

I deserve to be successful.

I am open to exciting new possibilities.

I am grateful for my talents and skills.

Wealth continuously flows through me.

Prosperity is my nature.

I am wealthy.

To get the most out of these affirmations, chant or listen to a recording every morning for 21 days. After this period, live with a more empowered and driven character. You can always return to these affirmations whenever you need to be reminded that you are abundant and successful.

Depression Affirmations

All your emotions are valid, and you have the right to feel them, including sadness. When you are sad, you keep thinking you will never be happy. But the truth is that happiness is always within reach. You are never short of reasons to be happy. These affirmations can help in uplifting yourself. This way, you will never go the route of depression.

I acknowledge my feeling of sadness.

I am allowed to feel all emotions freely.

The sadness that I feel is temporary.

I am willing to get past this feeling of sadness.

I am stronger than the sadness that I feel.

I let go of things that prevent me from being happy.

I am at peace with myself and everything else.

I let go of things I have no control over.

I invite peace and happiness.

I can see life's brighter side.

I acknowledge and recognize all my blessings.

I am grateful for all the blessings.

Today, I trust in the flow of life.

Life unfolds as it should.

Everything that I experience is for my own good.

Today, I take charge of my actions and feelings.

I live in the moment.

I have everything I need to feel happy.

I deserve to be happy.

I deserve all the good things in life.

I choose happiness.

Limitless happiness is my birthright.

My happiness comes from within me.

I uplift my happiness and the happiness of others.

I am feeling hopeful.

I believe that I can get through any problems in life.

I can solve any problems that I face.

I nourish myself with joyful food and kind words.

I am self-assured.

I am complete.

I am perfect despite my imperfections.

I am free of judgments that don't help me grow.

My blessings are greater than my fears.

What I can achieve is limitless.

I can do anything I set my mind to.

I am excited about all the opportunities that life is bringing to me.

Every opportunity in life takes me higher.

I am ready to pursue my dreams with certainty and passion.

Today, I take a step towards positive change.

My happiness is growing each day.

Always remember that it's okay to feel sad. The more important thing is learning to bounce back and find what makes you happy. Chant or listen to these affirmations if you are unhappy, extremely sad, or depressed. Listen to them for

21 days. After each practice, look into the world with brighter eyes and renewed hope that you will be happy.

Sexual Affirmations

As you get older, you learn more about how to rewire your brain. You can constantly remind your brain that you are okay, you are successful, you are happy, and you have a good sex life, even though you are still in the process of getting there or getting past the problems. This is what "fake it til you make it is about." You will tell yourself affirmations you want to hone and make yourself believe in them.

I am sexually appealing.

I embrace and explore my desires and passion.

I deserve sexual pleasure, and I consider it a gift.

I am full of passionate energy.

I am brimming with sexual confidence.

I am thankful for the sexual pleasures my body is giving me.

I engage in sexual behaviors according to my values.

I am in complete control of my sexual behaviors, feelings, and thoughts.

It's easy and natural for me to tell my partner what I want while making love.

My bed is my sanctuary where I feel sexually satisfied and safe.

It's easy for me to talk about sex with my partner.

My genitals are normal and healthy.

I have frequent and intense orgasms that satisfy my mind and body.

It always feels fun and exciting to get aroused.

My sex life is among the reasons why I am happy to be alive.

I am compassionate and patient about the sexual insecurities of my partner.

I remain humble and respectful when I get turned down by a potential sexual partner.

I am worthy of kindness and love from other people.

I treasure meaningful relationships by developing and maintaining them.

I show compassion and practice empathy for everyone, including myself.

I am complete whether I have a partner or not.

I am thriving emotionally and sexually.

I listen and pay attention to the needs of my body.

I can strongly sense my life's purpose.

As I explore my body, sexual wellness is becoming a priority.

Positive affirmations are helpful as long as they are part of a wider intervention technique. Make them part of your mindfulness practice, coaching, or therapy. You can't do affirmations without a goal. You will sound delusional if you only chant them without knowing why you're doing so. You will find it hard to believe what you are saying.

These are only samples of positive affirmations you can do as you try the other rapid weight loss strategies discussed in the next chapters. Remember to enjoy the journey. It is your body. It is your mind. It is your life.

You can set the pace and choose the techniques that work for you best.

In chapter one, I will brief you on why it is hard to lose weight and what your brain has to do with it. Once you are done with the affirmations, let's start learning more about hypnosis, emotional eating, your inner voice, and how all these are related.

CHAPTER ONE

Hypnosis Techniques to Help Lose Weight

Don't let the noise of others opinion drown out

your own inner voice.

- Steve Jobs

One of the hardest things to do in life is to lose weight. This is especially true when you've gone past your 30s. I know that feeling.

At this point, you will only get bigger if you do not focus on losing weight and maintaining whatever you have lost. But it's not easy. You have to sacrifice your favorite food and only allow for some cheat days just to make yourself feel like you are not being deprived. You must also make it a habit to wake up early, so you can exercise before starting your day.

Or you can get hypnotized.

HYPNOSIS AND WEIGHT LOSS

It's true; hypnosis and weight loss go hand in hand. First, you have to understand what hypnosis is about and what it is not.

I will try to go step-by-step to make it easier for you to understand the process. This is crucial since understanding is the first step toward connecting your physical manifestations, especially weight problems, to your mind's work.

If you have tried various weight loss programs before (with or without success for any reasons), you already have an idea of the backbone of all these programs - eat less and exercise more or burn more calories than how much to take in. If you do the opposite, the result will also be the opposite - you will gain weight.

This backbone of most exercise programs is the main reason they are bound to fail. They are too extreme in most cases that people would begin but would easily get discouraged to continue.

Additionally, diets that promote weight loss are too restricting most of the time. They prevent you from eating one or more food groups, portions, or food types too much and too fast. This will result in the feeling of deprivation.

Imagine eating your favorite food all your life, and in a blink of an eye, you are told that you cannot eat it anymore if you are serious about losing weight. It's like not seeing someone you loved without ever having a chance to say goodbye.

With the love sample, what will happen naturally is that you miss that someone. You would want to get back together the moment you see the person.

It is the same with food. You will crave it every day until the cravings become too much that you will suddenly find yourself binging at it one day without caring about your diet. When you reach this point, you will likely think hard about whether or not you would still go back to the restrictive diet. More often than not, people choose to be happy. They will eat whatever they want than go back to a diet program that will help them lose weight but will make them feel deprived or even depressed.

Aside from diet programs that feel too restricting, you will need to follow regular exercise programs. The exercises may start with simple routines, but they get more rigorous as you become more serious about your goal of losing weight and keeping your shape.

These exercises can leave you too weak since you are not eating much. If you cannot handle the pressure, you will eventually succumb to the stress. Instead of feeling rewarded for the weight you are losing, you will feel like being punished until the programs become more like self-inflicted suffering.

And you know in your mind that you can easily end that suffering when you stop following the diet and exercise programs. It's your choice.

I'm not telling you to quit dieting or doing rigorous exercises. But if they are doing more bad than good, you have to start weighing in what's more important. And that is whatever makes you happy.

WEIGHT LOSS FAILS

Do you ever wonder why you fail with your weight loss plans, no matter how intent you are? Why is it that when you think you've got everything right and under control, comes a bang and another failure after failure after failure?

Do you know that formula on how to lose weight?

As many fitness gurus have said, or maybe the science teachers you've had in the past, the fewer calories you take from the food and drink you take, the higher the chances you will lose weight.

In short, less calories, less mistakes.

While it's true and tested and a proven way to lose weight, it might also feel, at times, inhumane. You are restricting yourself from what it craves all the time. Because the minute you give in, you will gain back the cravings and the unwanted weight. And besides, the more you restrict yourself from eating, the more obsessed you become with food, which leads to hunger, irritability, and misery.

Animals in the wild eat what they want without getting overweight. You will only see overweight animals, with the ones captured and fed by humans. The animals in the wild eat to survive. They consume food to give them the energy to live. This is similar to human babies. They only cry and demand milk when hungry but stop sucking once they are full.

We were all once babies, so when did the problem begin? When did we start finding it difficult to stop eating and demanding even when our bodies tell us we're full?

The problem begins when we see food beyond its real purpose and no longer see it as something that will keep us alive. It starts to have different definitions and meanings. We begin to develop a relationship with food, which ignites a problem that will only get worse through time, especially if we don't set our feet firmly where we stand in this relationship.

As we nurture our relationship with food, we become psychologically attached to it. Once your unhealthy eating habits become ingrained in your mind, they will be hard to break and unlearn.

What now?

What will you do with a shapely body if you often feel depressed thinking about what you've been missing? These diets and exercises work. The only major problem is that they are hard to maintain.

You may be able to lose weight to fit into a dress for a special occasion, but after that day and you no longer have a goal, it might be harder to keep on depriving yourself of food while being enslaved with challenging exercises.

What you need is willpower. You have to convince your mind that you must start living healthy and find ways to adapt to a more active lifestyle.

The will has to come from you. It must be something that you badly want and not forced by anyone. Once you are convinced and have set your mind to the goal, you must begin breaking off the bad habits - the reasons why you gained and continue adding weight.

The easiest way to get this done is by saying goodbye to the bad habits and hello to the positive things and mindset you will bring as you go into weight loss hypnosis.

TAPPING INTO YOUR UNCONSCIOUS MIND

If you are serious about changing your "relationship" or your attitude towards food, the will to change must start from your unconscious mind.

Many people who have gotten into low points of their lives because of their weight issues ponder the same thing. Why can the diet industry not understand this complex relationship between people and food? Why do they keep coming up with diet plans that feel too restricting, often leading to failure?

The sad fact is that the diet industry is a booming business. That's how big of a problem being overweight is. It is a global problem. While there are diet plans with good intentions and don't merely want people to keep on buying their products after they've gotten back the weight they've lost, there are also those whose main goal is to profit from it all. However, the one thing they have in common is that they don't understand how the conscious and unconscious minds work as one in developing our eating behaviors.

This is where I will help you, and this is where you can use hypnosis to unlearn the unhealthy eating behaviors you have developed as you grow older.

I will help you tap into your unconscious mind until you finally realize how you ended this way. Your goal is to tap into your unconscious mind and complement the thoughts with what you consciously do. This will result in a positive change. This will help you lose weight more naturally, and this time, you will feel how rewarding the process is.

Before we delve further into the process, eliminate all the diet programs or pills you may have. They don't make you feel good about yourself. Most of the time, they make you feel happy. You no longer enjoy food like you used to, and they make you feel like you're always hungry.

What you need at the moment is something that will motivate you to change and adopt a healthier lifestyle, not because of a diet program but because this is what your heart and mind desire.

DEALING WITH YOUR WEIGHT ISSUES FROM YOUR CORE

Right this very moment, you have to commit. Be aware of your bad habits due to your complex relationship with food. What has led you to over-eat? When did you lose control of the portions of your food intake, and how many times did you eat?

It will help to keep a journal to record your progress. You can look back to this once you have successfully attained your goal of breaking the bad habits. Write in the journal every day. Consider it as your confidante who will listen to your thoughts, including the shame you find difficult to share with others.

Understanding the Emotions Brought about by Food

For the first part of your journal, start by listing the food you've consumed each day (morning, noon, lunch, and all the snacks in between). Parallel to the food names, you will write what you were feeling before eating the food. Were you stressed, bored, happy, upset, or angry that was why you've eaten the food or drank the beverage? Or were you feeling neutral, or you can no longer remember? Write them all down.

Be honest. This journal will help you realize that some of the bursts of hunger you feel at certain times during the day are habitual or emotional and no longer physical.

Understanding Emotional Eating

Habits develop over time, even without us realizing that they are becoming part of who we are. With the way you eat, you may not have planned it to become like this, but you have conditioned yourself to eat when you feel hurt, depressed, angry, or sad. We have various reasons for it, but we share something in common. There were points in our lives when food was used as a stimulus to elicit a response from us. Some of us may have been given treats by our parents when we were young to stop us from having tantrums or make our tears stop. And they do it every time we're in a bad mood or crying.

As we grow older, the stimulus/response behavior unwittingly taught by our parents becomes a habit that we cannot unlearn until the habit becomes harder to break. We seek food for comfort. We eat when we are in a bad mood. We eat to get rid of our pains.

When we eat in hopes of feeling better, but that does not happen, and instead, we feel worse, the tendency is to eat again. We will keep on eating until we get out of a negative or bad mood. Most of us have developed the habit of depending on sugar and sweets to get a temporary high. Sugar boosts our blood sugar levels, causing our mood to become happier and lighter. However, the high won't last. Afterward, your sugar levels will come crashing, and you'll feel worse again.

Our brains help in regulating our moods by keeping healthy levels of endorphins. However, the endorphins easily get depleted when we are faced with problems or exposed to much stress. When it happens, we instinctively think that we need a boost of endorphins, which we can get by eating something sugary or fatty. So then we will eat and feel better in a flash. After some time comes the realization that we've eaten something bad for our health, making us feel low again. It will become a cycle because we allow it to, even without intending it in the first place.

The journal will help you analyze the manner you eat or the pattern if you have already developed one. It may even make you realize that you already have habitual, compulsive eating, like eating when you're watching television or in the cinema or eating when you're bored.

Other unhealthy eating habits may have become your regular thing. These include eating something sweet or carbs whenever you have coffee or tea, finishing off the food offered to you at a party or someone else's place because you don't want to offend, or finishing off the leftover food of your children.

It's a good step to be aware of these habits. By making a journal about what you eat, when, why, and how you feel each time, you will realize that you have developed the habits and open your eyes to why you eat.

The following are the three common reasons why unhealthy people eat:

1. You are physically hungry.
2. Eating has become compulsive when you eat because you are emotionally hungry.
3. Eating has become a habit, so you do it even when you're not hungry.

Make these three reasons part of your journal. Mark each food you have eaten each day with the corresponding number that explains why you ate them.

This is your way of empowering yourself. You are now ready to discover the problem by becoming a witness to the habit or relationship you have developed with food. As you go about this day by day, you will become more aware. And by becoming aware, you can decide to change.

Write everything down in the journal. You ate this meal because you are physically hungry, and this is okay. But after you feel full but still eat something unhealthy, state why you did it. Was it because you were feeling stressed out at the time? If you did, what you have done was emotional eating. Or was it because it has become something innate that you will eat desserts or junk foods after your main meal. This is a sample of habitual eating.

Sometimes it would be hard for you to understand the reasons, so just write - I don't know, maybe I only got intrigued by how the food tastes like, or something like that. When you tap into your unconscious mind, the reasons for your compulsive eating behavior will be easier to understand. This is what we will deal with later on.

Listening to Your Inner Voice

At this point, you should already be aware of the reasons why you tend to overeat. These reasons will guide you in understanding the factors that led you to develop the behavior.

It's typical for everyone to develop a routine or the strategies they follow to be ready and do their everyday tasks. We all create a pattern of behavior according to how we react to triggers or stimuli. But it's not impossible to reprogram this behavior. No matter how old you are, you can teach your mind to adapt to new strategies.

This is where you need to listen to your inner voice. Relax and take a deep breath. Close your eyes and think or listen. If you feel like eating at this moment despite feeling full, listen to the voice. If you have only finished eating unhealthy food you told yourself to avoid, listen to the voice.

What does it say?

It's not surprising that the inner voice is scolding you, telling you truths, shaming your body, and shaming yourself. The inner voice tells you it is disgusted with what you have done or thought of doing.

Now imagine other people telling you the same things that your inner voice is nagging you at the moment. How would you feel? What if you are the one who is saying those words to someone you care about? How would you feel?

It's not good. The words hurt. You are not okay.

But you have to realize that the inner voice is you. Whatever you hear, whatever that inner voice says, is what you think about yourself. You are continuously berating yourself.

Why? Maybe you are disappointed, leading you to self-loathe and be caught between denial and reward. You have to stop the negativity. You have to realize that you are your worst critic, and you have been verbally abusing yourself all along. This has got to stop.

Change what that inner voice is saying by being kinder to yourself. By reading this book, you have already taken the first step towards freedom. You have taken the initiative to change and become better. And you are making a promise that you will do well. Praise yourself. Prompt the inner voice to say something positive to boost your confidence, and appreciate the good things you do for yourself and others.

Making Your Inner Voice Kinder

Go back to your journal and write. This time, you will write anything positive about yourself. You can write anything. It can be traits you are proud to have, something that other people told you, praise from a co-worker, a touching message from your child, and so on.

You will feed the inner voice with positivity. So write everything you want your inner voice to tell you the next time you try to listen to it.

Let me help you out by giving you samples.

"I always talk politely to others."

"I don't gossip."

"I am always there for my friends."

"I always lend a helping hand to a co-worker in need."

"I have beautiful eyes."

"I am a good child to my parents."

This is a practice of acknowledging all the good things about you. This will help you heal and love yourself more.

Now you are ready to make a commitment. You have to promise that you will change your relationship with food. From this day on, you will follow a healthier lifestyle.

Tell the inner voice that there will be bumpy roads ahead. You may not always feel positive and committed, but ask the voice to help you get back on track. Tell the inner voice to be patient and kind whenever you slip or have committed something unhealthy. Tell it to be supportive and encouraging. Tell it to yourself because the inner voice is you.

Making New Strategies

Habitual and compulsive eating behaviors are strategic. They were developed from our brains' instinct to work according to strategies. You resort to these behaviors because there was a trigger, an event or emotion in a familiar image or sound, recalled internal feeling, or a familiar internal dialogue. When you get the trigger, you can't help but do something you're accustomed to doing to gain something or complete the strategy. For example, you take a big bite of chocolate whenever you feel sad to feel comforted. You buy a bucket of popcorn when watching a movie at a theater house because it's part of the pattern.

At this time, you have to get rid of the old strategies and work on developing new ones. You can only change the strategy when you do it on your conscious and unconscious levels.

This is an exercise you need to follow to work on the triggers and change your response on a conscious level:

Think about a behavior you want to change. For example, reaching for a chocolate bar when you are sad. Focus on the situation you have chosen.

Keep your head down as you look to your left. Ask the inner voice what you want to change in this situation and tell it to show you how you would look after changing your behavior.

Now look up and look to your right. Imagine yourself having the new behavior and responding differently to the situation. As you imagine yourself becoming better and more positive, imagine that you're surrounded by people and notice their reactions.

Slowly bring your head down and look to your right. Imagine yourself walking away from the crowd. Look back and see what happened, like a film rolling right before your eyes. It's like seeing what change you have made, how other people react to it, how you looked and how it made you feel.

Do the exercise three times until you feel really good after coming out of the trance.

You will do this every time you are ready to turn a negative behavior into a positive one. The next time you do the exercise, get yourself first in your most relaxed position and close your eyes.

What you just did is help your mind form a strategy by thinking about the representation of the behaviors in feelings, sounds, and images. This way, you can reprogram and develop a new behavior that you will do next time a familiar trigger hits. After you have put all the patterns in place, they will become unconscious.

ENTERING INTO THE REALM OF HYPNOSIS

Unlike what many people believe, hypnosis can be done even without a medium. You can get into it even without the assistance of a hypnotherapist. You can perform a self-hypnosis, also referred to as focused thinking.

How do you get into a trance-like state?

Listen. All you have to do is to listen to recordings and follow what the voice says. This will help you change your strategies at an unconscious level.

This will unravel many answers, including the reasons why you fell into the trap of emotional or compulsive eating. This will make you realize when it was that you had developed a connection between feeling different and eating.

Many of your behaviors now as an adult come from past experiences regarding many aspects of your life. They include relationships, emotions, and events. Whatever you have gone through led to the formation of the connection between triggers and responses, which you have embraced because they make you feel happy and better. While you may be right at the time, whatever the causes and how you felt in the past might no longer feel the same at your age and where you are at the moment. When you were a child and finished all the food your mother prepared, you felt good because you knew she felt good for seeing that you appreciated her efforts to cook. But now that you've gone older and your metabolism slower, finishing your food, especially when you have a lot on your plate, makes you overweight.

As you can see in the sample, those were two similar behaviors at different points in your life. It made you feel happy when you were young, but you have the opposite feeling now that you are older.

What you need to do is to break the connection between how you feel and overeating, and you have to do it on an unconscious level. Achieving this will allow you to break free from the past behavior, move on, and start developing a healthier relationship with food.

What you need to understand now is the idea of a trance. It's like a floating feeling like you are daydreaming. It is a feeling you experience several times a day, but you are not only aware of when it happens. It's like the "in-between" feeling when you have just woken up from a deep sleep. It's like walking to the kitchen to drink water in the middle of the night, going back to bed, and not remembering what you did the early morning after you have fully woken up into consciousness. It's also similar to how a student feels when they study all night for an exam, walk to school during the day, and reach their destination without remembering how they got there.

You need focused thinking or give your full attention to reach the trance state. You can only get into that state after turning your attention inwards and allowing your unconscious mind to make the necessary changes without getting distracted by physical interruptions and the sound of your inner voice.

This is safe. You have nothing to get worried about. Even if you are in a trance state, you can switch back and become aware of your surroundings if you feel something urgent needs your attention.

Let's begin with self-hypnosis or focused thinking. You will find it beneficial to do this every day. Find a time when you know you won't be bothered, and you can have some alone time for yourself. This is a good practice to tap into your unconscious mind to make changes and destress.

What to do? Follow these steps:

1. Find a spot and get comfortable

Choose a spot where no one will bother you for 30 minutes or so. You have to feel comfortable and safe in it.

You can choose to lie down or sit, whatever feels more comfortable. Choose a spot above eye level where you will focus your gaze on.

Look at the spot with an intent gaze. Notice everything about the spot. As you do, notice what you are feeling and the sounds you hear. Breathe in deeply. As you slowly breathe out, look down until your eyes are closed.

Continue breathing deeply as you focus on how the air comes in and out of your body. Keep breathing deeply until the breathing becomes even and you become more relaxed. Focus on the relaxing feeling as you let it spread throughout your body to the point that you feel most comfortable, peaceful, and calm.

With your eyes still closed and you are breathing deeply, move your tongue to the top of your mouth. Allow your inner voice to be silent until you can no longer hear anything and get into a peaceful place inside your head.

Go to that peaceful place and imagine the texture and soothing colors filling it. Savor the feeling for a couple of minutes. Tell yourself congratulations because you are now ready to take control of your well-being for the days, months, and years to come.

Practice this first step until you have become a master of going into a peaceful place by silencing noises, including your inner voice. Once you have mastered this step, you can introduce situations when you reach a peaceful state.

2. Introducing situations during focused thinking

Your food journal will come in handy at this step. Go back to the times you were guilty of overeating. Choose one time, and focus on that while meditating.

Think about what you were doing that day, how you were feeling, and go back to the moment you saw the food you ate. Don't eat it this time. Instead, think about what you have done differently. Imagine yourself acting differently at that moment. Imagine what you feel, hear, and see.

Talk to yourself about the new attitude. Make sure you do it in a positive way. Tell yourself something positive about what you just did. For example, you can say - "I now see things objectively. I understand when I need to eat and when I want to eat. I now recognize when I am feeling emotional, and it's clear now that I don't have to rely on food when the emotions become overwhelming. I can overcome the feeling without eating, especially when I only want to eat but don't need it."

Now teach yourself about the affirmations you can return to whenever you are faced with a similar situation of feeling emotional and wanting to grab something to eat. Teach yourself how you can handle the situation better.

Here's an example of what you can tell yourself - "Every time I feel emotional, whether I'm stressed, upset, or angry, I will try to allow myself to calm down. I will close my eyes and focus on my breathing. I will think about what made me feel that way, and calmly, I will think of ways to handle things rationally, to get to the roots of the problem instead of finding temporary comfort from eating.

Once you have mastered the two mental exercises, you must find time to do both daily. Look into your food journal, and focus on a different reason or emotion you've experienced when you ate something unhealthy. One at a time. You can repeat similar emotions through the days if you think that you still have to grab a better grip of the emotions and yourself.

In a Nutshell

This chapter has introduced the usual reasons why weight loss programs fail, the main factor being most of them are too restricting.

- Instead of forcing yourself to cut down on food in a flash, you have to get to the bottom of things - the reasons why you are inclined to unhealthy eating and unhealthy food.
- Start a food journal to understand the pattern of what you're eating - when you do it because you need to and when you eat because you only want to. Understand the whys.
- Use your realizations on your first try in doing self-hypnosis.

CHAPTER TWO

Training Yourself to Eat When You Need It, Not When You Want It

The only time to eat diet food is while you're waiting

for the steak to cook.

- Julia Child

In this chapter, you will teach yourself to have a more natural and rewarding relationship with food. You will learn how to take charge of your thoughts and actions. Your goal here is to feel pleasure when you eat and not guilt.

TRAINING YOURSELF TO EAT WHEN YOU'RE PHYSICALLY HUNGRY

You may have unintentionally trained yourself to feed your emotional hunger that you may no longer remember the last time you were physically hungry. If you have resorted to diet programs without feeding your physical hunger, your body may have trained itself into thinking that you have deprived it of food. As a result, it stored fat to hold on to the calories, which made you fat.

This is why training yourself to eat only when you feel physically hungry is important.

But how will you know that you are indeed physically hungry?

There are four stages of hunger. Before grabbing food, you have to check every hour or two in which category your level of hunger falls into:

1. Not hungry at all
2. There's a slight twinge of hunger
3. Hungry, and I want to eat now
4. Very much hungry that I can eat a bear if I see one

This is how your physical hunger progresses. So when do you eat? It is best to grab something when you hit C. Don't wait until D because being too hungry will make you eat more than you should. And more often than not, when you reach D, you will likely grab any food you see, including the unhealthy ones.

Make it a habit to check in which stage your hunger is in. The more you get used to it, the quicker you will get accustomed to it. There will come a time when you no longer need to check because it will be easier to pinpoint when your hunger is at a C.

If you still aren't used to reading signals, there will be times when your body may confuse thirst with hunger. You can deal with this by ensuring your thirst won't interfere with your hunger. To get this done, drink about an ounce of water per hour. You can drink more if you want. Water is generally beneficial and will help your body function naturally. It helps by boosting your metabolism and flushing out toxins.

When you eat because you're hungry, remember to stop eating at once when you no longer feel the hunger. Stop even if you haven't tasted the dessert or you are being offered another serving of your favorite dish.

Stop eating when you are pleasantly full. Do not wait until you feel uncomfortable or stuffed. You also must train yourself to recognize when you have satisfied your physical hunger. This will take time to retrain your thoughts to recognize when you are full. Typically, your body sends you a signal when you are full and need to stop eating. But more often than not, we override the signal until it comes to the point that we no longer remember what this signal is. At this moment, you have to train yourself to recognize and notice the signal when it is present.

A good way to train yourself to recognize the signal is by eating slowly. This is also referred to as mindful eating. When you eat, you will focus on the food - the taste, the smell, and the texture. You will also focus on how you chew the food and make sure that you only swallow once you have chewed thoroughly and slowly. You will focus on how it makes you feel.

Doing mindful eating regularly will make it easier to recognize signs that you are full over the days. Eating usually begins with a pleasurable feeling. You must notice when the pleasure begins to subside, meaning you enjoy your food less. This is your signal to stop eating.

Do not feel bad if you have food leftovers on your plate. It will make you feel worse if you force yourself to finish everything and feel bad afterward. To avoid leftovers, use a smaller plate next time. You can also add food to your plate a little at a time.

Make It a Sensory Experience

Emotional eating has deprived you of enjoying food for what it is. Now you are ready to make eating a pleasurable experience. You can now focus on feeling pleasure because you have broken the connection between habit and emotion. But before moving forward, make yourself this promise - "I will only eat when I am certain that it feels pleasurable to eat."

Most of the time, dieting also takes away the pleasure of eating. It limits your calorie intake and pushes you to consume meal replacements. More often than not, the meal replacements no longer taste natural or can even be tasteless. As a result, you only eat for the sake of it and to continue functioning, but you have already taken away the pleasure from eating.

You need to taste your food to feel pleasure and appreciate what you're eating. Dieting involves chemicals and artificial sweeteners to be added to your food. The truth is our bodies find it harder to break them down. Instead of focusing on breaking down your fat intake and converting it to energy, your system has to deal with the chemicals. In the long run, the unnatural substances don't help in trimming you down. But instead, they result in the opposite.

You have to make eating an experience, and not just any experience but something great and pleasurable.

What do you do?

From now on, take pleasure in preparing natural food. Choose healthy ingredients and prepare them in ways you and your family will enjoy. Stop eating processed food, artificial sweeteners, or restricting yourself from reduced calorie, low-fat, and other diet fads.

Learn to appreciate food's natural flavors and taste by eating and chewing slowly. Also, eat only when you know that you will take pleasure in eating. Eat when you are truly hungry because that is when you will appreciate the appearance, smell, texture, and flavor of what you are eating.

Always eat because it's time to eat, not when you're sad or bored. When eating, pay attention to how you are feeling. Stop at once when you are full.

You also have to start exploring new foods. Create new meals and combine flavors. You need to develop an interest in tasting something new.

Why do you need to lose weight?

It is your way of telling your body - "I respect you." In doing so, you will become less prone to sickness, have clearer eyes and skin, gain more energy, and become healthy in general.

Taking a Stand

Now that you are en route to a healthier you, making healthier choices in food and eating the right portion only when it's time to eat, how do you deal with temptations?

Your relationship with food may have changed, but bear in mind that other people may not see it that way. Despite your obvious struggles, families and peers will still invite you to dine out, parties, BBQs, coffee, and other meetups or events where you might be forced to eat more than you need when you are not feeling hungry.

But you don't have to give in. You can still come with them, but it is your option to eat or not or eat only the portions that will suit your newfound relationship with food.

This may be easier said than done. I understand. We often feel like we're being impolite if we will refuse the host's extra serving of their specialty or to have a dessert or try something bought by a friend.

When you feel like you'd be impolite to say no, remember your struggles to be at a state where you can control your eating pattern. Politely refuse and be truthful about the reasons. You will be surprised to know that people would be understanding of your situation. Many will even admire you for your will to become healthier and may even compliment you on losing weight. Some will also get curious about how you did it.

It is always your choice. You can say no when you want. You can have coffee at the coffee shop without ordering a slice of cake. You can attend a party serving a buffet without filling your plate with all the dishes.

However, if you really fancy a piece of cake or you are Stage C hungry, then eat. You don't have to be too restricting to yourself. But be mindful of the signal when your body tells you it is full. Remember to stop eating when the process stops feeling pleasurable.

What about when you are eating in a restaurant where the serving sizes are too much? If you have a companion, you can ask them beforehand if they can share the food with you. If they refuse or if you are eating alone, you can ask the server if you can order food in half servings. If not, just tell them to bring you half servings, and you will pay in full (or ask the half to be packed to go).

The idea here is to find ways to be resourceful on how you will talk your way out of the possibility of overeating.

HYPNOSIS MEDITATION TO GET INTO A RESOURCEFUL STATE

Your goal for this meditation is to get yourself into the right state. The process is similar to how you do focused thinking. Before starting, make sure you go to a quiet spot where you can't be bothered while meditating.

Relax and make yourself comfortable. Breathe deeply until you're feeling ready to begin.

Close your eyes. Think about the time when you felt powerful and full of determination and confidence. Take your time thinking about the moment where you will focus on. Whether it's a memory several years back or something you have experienced recently, it doesn't matter.

If you can't think of a time or experience in your life when you felt too powerful and in control, you can think of another person. Think of someone who has the qualities that you want to embody. This person may be someone you admire.

After choosing the experience (or person), focus on what happened at the time when you felt determined (or how the person you admire reacted to a situation that made you think they are determined).

Focus, and notice all the things about the experience - what are you wearing, what happened, what did you say, how other people responded, how they looked, and how you felt.

Make the picture bigger. Make it clearer. Imagine as if you can hear everything louder. Keep on focusing, and make the situation more perfect. Change the things you want to change, or add an event, people, or something you could have said or done better until the scenario feels perfect.

Step into the scene, and feel like you are really there in the scenario. See through your eyes, and feel like you are there. Experience the feeling of being there - like the scene unfolds before you. Let the feeling of being confident grow as your determination grows until you feel powerful. Savor the experience until you feel like you are in control.

Make a fist with your right hand. Focus on the feeling as you squeeze it tight. The more you squeeze, the more powerful, confident, and determined you feel. Gently release the fist. Open your eyes and close them right away.

Now you will imagine something that will happen in the future. You will focus on a scenario where people are persuading you to eat more. Or they keep on insisting you add more food to your plate. Like a scene from a movie, freeze the frame. You see yourself and the other people in the scene more clearly.

What are you seeing? It can be a relative who insists you try their freshly-baked cake or have more if you already had a bite. You may be standing at a buffet table with your friends who keep adding food to your plate while saying that you must try this and that.

Now walk into the scene as the movie starts playing again. Instead of witnessing things happening, be there. Feel like you are in the scene, and you are seeing and hearing everything as they happen. Make a fist in your right hand and squeeze it tight. As you do, let yourself feel the surge of strength, determination, and confidence. Be there, and politely refuse foods you know you can't eat. Tell them why.

Make them understand that you are already full. Linger on how it feels to be in control. And see the look of admiration from those who have witnessed what happened. Hear what they are saying. Hear your own words. Did you laugh as you refuse and tell them this is the new you? Did you feel lighthearted and accomplished? Did the other people in the scene smile after hearing what you said? Savor the carefree feelings, the smiles, the laughter, the acceptance. As you release your fist, open your eyes.

In a Nutshell

You have learned how to develop a rewarding relationship with food - to make the experience pleasurable instead of feeling guilty when you overeat.

- The chapter listed the four stages of hunger - not hungry, slightly hungry, physically hungry, and very much hungry.

- Make sure that you only eat when you are physically hungry, but don't wait until you are very much hungry because it will push you to overeat, which will make you feel guilty.
- From now on, you will not only enjoy the food but the process. You will begin practicing mindful eating.
- Chew your food slowly, and experience the process. Taste the food and notice how it makes you feel. As you do, wait for your body's signal when it's full and stop eating once it hits you.
- Lastly, practice the hypnosis meditation that will help you get into a resourceful state. Do it nightly until you have mustered the courage and confidence to tell other people that you can't overeat.

CHAPTER THREE

Taking Your Relationship with Food to the Next Level

It is like whispering to one's self and listening

at the same time.

- Mina Murray about journaling

(in Bram Stoker's Dracula)

You have already started with healthy changes that will serve as important groundwork for your future relationship with food. This chapter will help you work on that future with a new lifestyle and satisfying, sustainable, and successful changes.

The future begins today.

It's an evolving process filled with success, but expect challenges along the way. It all begins by creating your future, which is different from setting goals.

You are not going to set goals to achieve in weeks, months, or years from now. What will happen after you have successfully attained them all, or what if you don't? This kind of goal setting only works for sports, studies, or business. It's different when you want to set something for personal progress or triumphs.

You have to create your future every day. This is the beginning of your journey to a happier and healthier lifestyle. You will carry this with you for the rest of your life.

Each day starting today, you will visualize yourself as a sculptor perfecting a healthier and slimmer you. You will see progress every day. The changes may be gradual, but they will make you proud.

In creating your future, make sure that you focus on these two factors:

- Think that your future is going to be positive. Focus on the things you want to achieve, and do not dwell on anything you don't want to happen.
- You have all you need to make things happen, enforce big life changes, and start leading the life you want. The changes are bound to happen starting today.

Bring out your journal.

Write everything that comes to your mind about what you want to happen in your future. How do you envision yourself, and what do you want your life to be like? Write about what you think the impacts you're doing today will have on yourself, the things you do, and others.

MEDITATION IN CREATING YOUR FUTURE

Go to your quiet spot, and be comfortable. Close your eyes as you prepare yourself for another meditation. This time, you will focus on creating your future.

Visualize a line. Imagine this line as your life. Whatever is in front of the line is your future, and what's beyond it is your past.

Now float above the line. Look at it to see your life below you.

Look into your future, and visualize yourself being healthy and strong on your 80th birthday.

See the look of contentment and how happy you are. This is what you have become after having lived a life free from criticism, self-doubt, and compulsive eating. This is who you have become after turning your back on unhealthy ways and old habits.

Float and go to the scene in your future. Imagine yourself being at the scene. You are right there, celebrating your 80th birthday while feeling like you are at your best. Be there. See everything. Hear and feel everything. This is your ideal future, so savor the moment.

Now start traveling to the present - to your life at the moment. Don't rush, so you can experience every step of the way. As you travel, stop every time a moment hits that you want to cherish. You don't have to remember what the moment exactly is. You only need to relinquish the feeling. You will need them to create your ideal future.

Once you get into your present, imagine a thing that connects the present you to the future you. It can be a rope, thread, or ribbon of any color, size, and texture. Aside from serving as a connection, this thing will be your guide to your journey in realizing the future you've created.

STAY POSITIVE

No matter how hard you try to keep your mind focused on positive thoughts and beliefs, there will come a time when that inner voice will interfere. It will bring back the beliefs you still haven't gotten rid of completely. And these beliefs would hold you back.

From now on, always go back to the thought that the best way forward is to stay positive. Do your best to silence self-doubt. If there is still a part of you that doesn't believe you can make the changes permanently, silence the doubts and remind yourself you can do it, and you will succeed no matter what.

WRITING ACTIVITY - BRING OUT YOUR JOURNAL

In your journal, you will write down all your self-doubts. Think hard about the things, thoughts, or people that stop or slow down your progress at the time when you thought that you were on your way to a healthier you.

Here are some samples:

My mother said I'd be fatter anyway when I get older because it runs in the genes.

I am always a failure with whatever I do. Why would I make an effort to lose weight when I'd fail myself eventually?

I may not be able to resist when all my friends go on an eating spree without feeling sorry for myself.

What you have listed are your old beliefs that you need to get over with. It will be easier to accomplish when you change them.

Beliefs are bound to change as you get older. When you were younger, you used to believe in Santa Claus, the Tooth Fairy, or you needed to get married by the time you reached the age of 30, and so on.

What happened? You find out most of these beliefs are not true as you become older and wiser. There are also certain beliefs that you have found a better option for when you have gotten older.

This is also your goal with the limiting beliefs that slow your progress to become fitter and healthier.

No Buts

The best way to test your commitment to the goal of changing your future is to hear your response to relevant questions. Are you fully committed to changing the habits that are making you fat? Or is there a part of you that keeps saying "but?"

Do you still answer questions like - "A part of me says yes, but..."? If this is the case, then you have to be more determined. It's understandable that a part of you remains protective - the part that has seen you disappointed and unsuccessful with your previous goals. Both parts of yourself may agree on certain points at a time, but when self-doubt becomes too much to bear, the protective side will win.

How do you delete the buts in your explanations? You have to work hard to combine the two parts of your personality. Your goal is to have only one answer whenever there is a question, which is a positive answer with no buts.

MEDITATION TIME - RESOLVING YOUR INNER CONFLICT

This meditation aims to combine the two conflicting parts of how you think. This will focus on the positive intentions and try to resolve the contradictory thoughts.

Go to your quiet spot and be at your most comfortable. Shut all noises from around you because you need to focus on what your inner thoughts will say.

First, you need to pinpoint what it is that you want to triumph on and why you are having such a hard time doing so.

You have to learn to identify when the two parts of yourself are making the decision instead of one.

For example, "I want to prepare my own healthy foods at home from now on. But I'm busy, so it will be hard to do it every day."

You have to catch yourself whenever you think that way, which means that the two sides of your personality are talking - the motivated and the doubtful.

What do you do?

You will give each personality a face. Place each of them in each of your hands. You need to imagine how they look and how they sound. Imagine them saying the words to you, one being motivated and the other doubtful. Imagine what emotions are connected to each.

Now put your palms up and let them face you. Imagine that you are confronting these two sides of you. Ask each of them what they want to say.

In the given example, your motivated part might say, "You will find joy in learning healthier recipes and the creative ways you can prepare them." Whereas the other part would say, "You are busy, and preparing your own healthy food from scratch might stress you out. I only want you to keep things simpler."

Talk to them and continue hearing what they have to say. They both have valid reasons. They only want what's best for you. One part wants you to be healthier, and the other doesn't want you to feel the added burden.

Allow them to talk some more. It will take time before they come into an agreement, but hear everything they're saying. Once you feel like you've heard enough, thank both parts for their contribution. Then, ask them to form a powerful combination with the utmost positive intention for you.

Slowly, bring both hands together. Intertwine your hands and feel the joining of the two forces. Pull your hands close to your heart as if you are taking these two parts of you back inside, but this time, they are one.

Relish the feeling before coming out of a trance. You can also combine this with other meditations to make it easier to imbibe the positive and gradually release all the negativity within.

GUIDED MEDITATION TO STOP EMOTIONAL EATING

This guided meditation will help you deal with emotional eating by facing the problem. It is time to accept that there really is a problem, and you are ready to confront it.

Before beginning this meditation, find a quiet space or a spot where you will remain unbothered for several minutes.

Choose an area where you are comfortable and where it feels at home.

Make yourself physically, mentally, and emotionally comfortable. You can sit or lie down, whatever you prefer. Relax all parts of your body, and close your eyes. Relax your lungs and pay particular attention to your heart chakra.

Eliminate all thoughts as much as possible to allow your mind to relax. Forget about the worries at this moment and relax.

Breathe, Be Comfortable, and Breathe

Breathe deeply through your nose. Hold it for two counts.

Release your breath slowly.

Breathe deeply through your nose for the second time, and hold it for a count of two.

Gently release the breath.

Continue breathing deeply in your most comfortable and peaceful position as you take in the following words. Think about all these thoughts about emotional eating. Take this time to recognize the problem, understand its roots, and help yourself heal, recover, and move forward.

Remind yourself that you have nothing to prove. No one is forcing you to do anything. But this is the sacred time you wish to spend to focus on yourself - your feelings, thoughts, and body. This is your time to be with the real you - your authentic self.

Use this meditation to confront whatever has been instilled into the innocent subconscious mind that made you believe over the years that you don't have control over your eating.

You know in yourself that you feel ashamed. You don't know to whom or what, but you feel shame due to emotional eating.

Take this moment to accept the shame and forgive yourself for doing it, for losing control, and for allowing yourself to continue doing it even after seeing what it is doing to your body and overall health.

Accept that it's not your fault that after allowing yourself to resort to emotional eating once, it has become a habit you can't control. It is not your fault that you have found comfort in emotional eating. For as long as you allowed it to last, it has brought you relief from spiritual starvation.

Now you have to accept that emotional eating has nothing to do with physical hunger. It has nothing to do with food.

A different kind of hunger causes emotional eating. You resort to it due to spiritual hunger and starvation.

Forgive the Inner Child

Do not blame yourself if food has become a friend. In most cases, food addictions start from childhood. Children who are extremely lonely, who often feel alone and abandoned, turn into food to take away the loneliness or emptiness filling them, not knowing that what they are filling is not physical but spiritual hunger.

If you are that child, forgive that child. It is not that child's fault that it has developed a deep relationship with food; you had treated food as your only friend back when you were young.

You must confront the patterns by understanding them logically and cognitively.

When we suffer from food addiction of any kind, we go through a roller coaster ride of emotions; hence, we eat for emotional reasons.

You start with the beginning rooms - the rooms that make you reach out for food. Then the emotions come into play. You eat and then, later on, blame yourself.

After the blame came the shaming part. You feel ashamed of your weight. You feel shameful for your physical appearance and your behavior.

You have this wound, the original one, rooted in feeling not good enough.

Growing Older with the Habit and an Unhealed Wound

As you get older, since you did not do anything to know what had caused the problem or where the pain was coming from, you continue with the habit of relying on food for comfort.

Through time, the behavior reinforces the unhealed wound - that pain, which reminds you, no matter how hard you try to set aside, that you are not good enough.

You have to begin understanding that even though your emotional eating is rooted in a deep, unhealed wound or many painful wounds, there is only one way to free yourself from unhealthy patterns.

Open yourself up to the idea that your habits are reinforcing the wounds you thought would heal on their own but did not.

Think about the innocent child. That was you. The wounded child turned to the food instead of confronting the wound. As a result, the child developed a pattern of emotional eating to get comforted.

This is no one's fault. This is not the child's fault. You are not the villain. No one is. It is a matter of programming and patterns.

Your brain has learned to associate pleasure with eating by turning onto food to feel comforted. This pattern is easy for your brain to understand since food easily affects your mood.

Usually, when we feel lonely, the instinct is to reach out for foods high in saturated fats, salt, and carbohydrates. After feasting on these foods, our brain feels good.

This is the start of a pattern. When you allow it to happen often, your brain will associate the pleasurable feeling with eating unhealthy foods.

Your brain wants to help you. It doesn't want you feeling the pain. When you are feeling down, your brain instinctively knows that food will perk you up and lighten your load.

This is no longer a choice of whether you will do it or not. This is already biology and chemistry.

Best of all, bear this in mind. This is not your fault.

But you can still do something to break the pattern by understanding first and foremost how your brain works. Understand that your brain would always want you to avoid pain, and it always acts to help you attain that.

PREPARING FOR THE HINDRANCES ALONG THE WAY

The journey toward losing weight is not easy. You will face obstacles no matter what you do or how determined you are. Everything around you will have an impact on your journey to a healthier you - your work, relationships, friends, and daily life. They will influence your journey positively and negatively at some point in your life.

Some hindrances will be easy, and some will be demanding or stressful. This is what you need to watch out for. Ensure that you don't fall into the trap of stress. You have to identify stress once it is present and deal with the cause at once.

Allowing stress to beat you might lead you to go back to your old habits of resorting to food. You have already done a lot. Now is not the time to quit just because life has become pretty stressful.

Stress is common, and there are many ways to deal with it. Let's expound on the subject in the next chapter.

In a Nutshell

In this chapter, you have made steps in taking your relationship with food to another level.

- You have envisioned yourself as a sculptor that continuously makes a masterpiece - your body.
- Your goal is to make progress with your artwork each day. And you will write everything in your journal.
- You have also learned how to meditate in creating your future. You have seen the healthy and fit version of yourself celebrating your 80th birthday.
- The sight has made you proud, and this motivates you to bring a connection with that future to your present self.

- In your journal, you will write down all your self-doubts. You will also realize the times when you always say the word "but."
- You will recognize the two parts inside you - the one that motivates and the one that is overprotective and always says but.
- By meditating, you will try to resolve the conflicts between these two sides of you. You will hear them out and, in the end, combine the two.
- Your goal is to stay positive as much as you can.

You also need to recognize that there will be hindrances along the way. Most of them will be caused by stress. Let's delve more into this in the next chapter.

CHAPTER FOUR

Learn How to Deal with Everyday Stress

You are braver than you believe, stronger than you seem,

and smarter than you think.

- Christopher Robin (in A.A. Milne's Winnie the Pooh)

Stress is the main reason why you resort to emotional eating. It makes you want to reach out for anything you can eat to get comforted at once. But it doesn't have to be always like that. You have to learn what stress is and how to effectively deal with it to avoid overeating whenever you're stressed out.

Remember that stress is not always bad. It only becomes unhealthy when it becomes too much to the point that you are becoming frustrated.

Stress is how your body reacts to anything it sees as a threat. The cause of stress is called a stressor.

What happens is that when your system feels a sudden demand or threat, your nervous system floods your body with stress hormones to help you cope. These hormones, including adrenaline and cortisol, prompt you to take action. They make your heart beat faster and your blood pressure higher. However, it also makes you more aware of your surroundings by making your senses sharper.

When your body feels the tension due to stress, you become more focused. You also feel stronger, which makes you do things faster than usual. Once your body feels threatened, it will automatically go into the flight or fight response. This is your body's way of protecting you, which becomes helpful in an emergency.

There are instances when it can save your life. For example, when you are driving and a person crosses the street out of the blue. You will immediately slam on the brakes to avoid the accident. What prompted you to take action is the feeling of stress. It alerts your mind and helps keep your focus and remember what to do.

Another good thing about stress is that it helps you get over your fear. It keeps your mind focused and sharp. For example, stress makes you feel motivated if you have stage fright but a presentation to do. You will study and prepare to ensure you won't make a fool of yourself at the time of the presentation.

Stress becomes bad when it starts affecting your mind and body negatively. When it becomes too much and happens too often, your body can no longer recognize the real threats. As a result, it enters into a fight or flight mode over and over again.

When this happens, you become vulnerable to emotional and mental attacks. You also become vulnerable to health concerns, including the following:

- Heart ailments and stroke
- Depression
- Digestive issues
- Muscle pains
- Sleep disorder
- Skin problems
- Lower immunity
- Weight disorders

STRESS AND FOOD

Turning to food is one of the unhealthiest ways of dealing with stress. People eat even when they are not hungry. They eat more than what they can take in. They binge on food but do not have the energy to exercise.

On the other hand, there are also those with the opposite reaction to stress and food. They tend to skip eating when stressed. They lose their appetite and do not eat even when they are hungry.

Both these responses to stress are unhealthy. You can either gain weight or lose weight fast.

THE ROOTS OF STRESS

Knowing where it is coming from is the best way to deal with the problem. Stress can be due to different factors and can affect people differently.

Here's a look at the most common causes of stress:

1. Feeling like there is a demand to step up

This is something that can be looked into positively and negatively. You are stressed when faced with a deadline, a tight schedule, or when you undergo difficult phases in your relationship.

You feel stressed when you are undergoing positive events. They include getting married, having a child, buying a new house, studying college, or starting a new job.

2. Other people's influence

Your behavior is often a result of the attitude of the people you surround yourself with. However, it can also be stressful when you are alone and isolated. The lack of human interaction can trigger stress. If you have to choose a company, it is best to keep a pool of positive and happy individuals. Hang out with people who cheer you whenever life's a mess and those who will be there through ups and downs.

3. External factors

External factors that can trigger stress include financial and relationship problems. It can be caused by major changes in the family, work, and social aspects of life. It can also be due to the feeling you are always running out of time.

4. Internal factors

These are the self-generated factors leading to more worries, pessimism, and becoming irrational. They include being a perfectionist, having too many expectations, and having difficulty adjusting to sudden changes in plans.

DEAL WITH STRESS USING YOUR SENSES

You have to learn how to deal with stress every day. You can't perfect the skills overnight, so you must keep improving every day. The best way to do this is to utilize your senses.

Here's a look at how to use your senses in dealing with stress:

Sense of sight

It is best to surround yourself with images and things you can look at whenever you feel stressed. They can be anything that will help you feel better and lighter. You can put pictures of your loved ones at your office desk, or bring outdoor elements inside, such as flowers and plants. You can also add elements to your surroundings in colors that you find relaxing. If you have time, you can take a quick stroll to enjoy the view while trying to feel calmer.

If you don't have any material things to look at or can't go someplace, you can use your imagination and visualize images that will help you unload the heaviness.

Here's a quick meditation you can do using your sense of sight to deal with stress. If you can't go to a quiet spot, just close your eyes and try to minimize or completely shut off the noise from your surroundings:

With your eyes closed, allow your mind to take you to your favorite place. It can be anywhere - your favorite spot in the house, park, or beach. Relax while imagining you are walking. See the beauty surrounding you, and enjoy the view.

Sense of hearing

Try alleviating your stress by focusing on your auditory sense. There are many things you can do, and see which one will lift your mood.

You can listen to relaxing music or sing your favorite song. It will also help to hang a wind chime near you or put a miniature fountain at your work desk to enjoy its soothing sounds when you're agitated.

If you have time, you can go to the park or beach and settle in a spot where you feel safe and comfortable. Sit and close your eyes. Listen closely to the sounds of nature. This is your chance to appreciate the sound you tend to ignore. They include the waves' coming and going, chirping birds, the rustling of the wind, and more.

You can also meditate to get rid of stress using your sense of hearing. This is best for those who are tone deaf or can't sing, or you can also do this if you can't go someplace else to listen to calming sounds. This is called vocal toning.

To begin the meditation, you must sit up straight and be comfortable. You will start making sounds like how it's done in yoga. Say "hmm" as you listen intently. Say it repeatedly while changing the speed, volume, and pitch. Check how your body responds to the changes in how you say the hum. Repeat the sound that makes you feel the calmest.

Sense of smell

This is recommended for people who freeze, get stoned, or feel disoriented when stressed. Your goal is to find the scent that soothes you and helps in calming your nerves. Look for scents with invigorating and energizing effects.

You can also do the following to check which scent suits you best in dealing with stress:

- Burn an incense or light a scented candle
- Dab your favorite perfume or cologne on your cloth
- Smell the flowers
- Step outside and smell the fresh air

- Add some drops of essential oil to your shampoo. This way, you will smell the scent throughout the day as it remains in your hair
- Use a lavender-scented fabric conditioner on your bed sheets and pillowcases

Sense of touch

Using your sense of touch, you will start feeling things your skin gets in contact with. Feel the texture and focus on the feelings that the materials bring about. Through this, you will know the textures and materials you can feel or wear whenever you are stressed.

Here are some of the things you can do:

- Soak in a hot bath and linger on how you feel as the water hits your skin. You may want to add several drops of your favorite essential oil to the water to use your sense of smell and touch at the same time.
- Have a massage. You can do this yourself, but it will be better to have someone else do it for you, especially when you want a full-body massage. But having any massage will do, such as hand, back, or neck.
- Play with your pet and touch their body and fur.
- Wear anything that makes you feel lighter and comfortable. Choose something that feels great on the skin when worn.

Sense of taste

This is still part of the mindful eating process. You will indulge in your food but not overeat. Focus on the food's taste and how they make you feel as you slowly chew on them. While doing this, make sure that you keep everything in moderation. Always remind yourself that you are doing all these to lose weight and maintain that shape. You are taking every step to become healthy and refrain from retracing your steps to an unhealthy lifestyle.

You already know how to do mindful eating, but here are some quick stress relief tips you can follow:

- Slowly sip your favorite hot or cold drink. It can be a steaming cup of tea, coffee, iced juice, or soda. It can be your favorite wine. Whatever you decide to drink, sip it slowly and indulge in the taste.
- Have a bite of dark chocolate and let it linger on your tongue. Feel its texture and focus on the taste.
- Munch on healthy snacks, like sliced carrots, celery, or fruits.
- Pop a sugarless gum in your mouth and chew it slowly.

Sense of movement

If your initial reaction to stress is by freezing or shutting down, you have to utilize your sense of movement when stressed out. This reaction is typically seen in those who have undergone trauma. Since you already know how your body will respond to stress, beat the reaction. Move your body before it freezes or before you feel agitated and unable to move.

Here are some of the things you can do to beat stress using your sense of movement:

- Stretch your body and flex your muscles
- Jog into place
- Jump up and down
- Dance
- Squeeze a stress ball
- Go for a short walk outside

QUICK STRESS RELIEF IN THE MOMENT TECHNIQUES

It is not uncommon to get caught by stress when you least expect it. Learning how to deal with stress effectively doesn't come overnight. It takes practice, but as long as you do them every time you deal with stress, everything will fall into place eventually.

Take it easy, and start small. You can take one step at a time and reward yourself every time you successfully deal with it.

You can also try verbalizing how you feel. It will help to talk to someone about what you are going through. You will be amazed at how many people will reach out and can relate to what you're going through.

Here are six easy techniques you can do to try and relieve yourself from stress the moment it hits you:

1. Laugh

You may have heard a thousand times before that laughter is the best medicine. And it's true, even when you force yourself to do it. Try laughing out loud whenever stress is beating you down. Laugh even without reason. To make it easier, you can try remembering a funny joke, something you've watched on TV, or a funny situation you've witnessed.

It may sound unnatural initially, especially when forcing yourself to laugh, but don't stop. As you laugh and hear yourself laughing, you will recall funny moments that will make you laugh harder. Laughing is an exercise that relaxes your muscles and helps release endorphins in the brain.

2. Body scan meditation

This meditation will help you become aware of your body sensations. To do this, you have to go to your quiet spot and sit and lie comfortably. Close your eyes and shut off the noises around you. Focus on your core and prepare as you begin mentally scanning your different body parts.

Begin on your left foot. How does it feel? Move it as you mentally scan the body part. If you feel any tension, use the power of your mind to ask the stress to go away.

Continue with the process with each body part up to your head. Whenever you encounter tension, bring in the power of your mind and tell the source of tension, which is stress, to go away.

This meditation can be finished in ten minutes or less. You can end it by focusing on the now - bring your focus to the present time. Breathe deeply as you open your eyes. Rejoice as you imbibe the benefits you have gained from the meditation you just did.

3. Dance

Dancing is good for your body. It's a form of exercise that release and pump up your endorphins. It doesn't have to be grand, and you can do it without bothering anyone with the music or your movements. You can do it somewhere you are alone, like your room, garden, or in the bathroom.

You can begin by putting on your earphones to hear the music. Dance even if you are not good at it, and dance as if nobody's watching. Continue to dance even when there are other people around. You will notice how it makes you feel better and happier as you beat your fear of being caught dancing by other people. If you are doing it in the office and your co-workers see you and they smile, think about it as an accomplishment. In your own way, you have made other people's stress a little lighter.

4. Listen to nature

Listening to nature is a good way to remind yourself of the bigger world; you may have problems, but it's not the end. If you are undergoing a difficult phase in your life, remember that this will pass. Life will move on, and it will become better.

When stressed, try to calm your nerves so you can think clearly. You can do this exercise indoors or outdoors. If you are in the office and have a break, use the time to go somewhere like a park and sit on a bench. Close your eyes and listen to the nature that surrounds you. It can be the whistling of the air and leaves as they move, animals making sounds, listening to any sound in your environment, and listening intently.

As you listen, imagine yourself someplace where you see the source of the sounds. Make this place idyllic and satisfying. You can be anywhere your mind takes you. It can be a beach, the mountains, a camping site in the wild, or anywhere you like. Listen to the sounds while envisioning yourself in different surroundings. Allow yourself to get comforted and soothed.

You can also use your phone to do this. You can download apps that allow you to play nature sounds accompanied by nature photos or videos. Nature sound tripping will help a lot to refrain your system from producing stress hormones.

5. Practice deep breathing

A minute of this breathing exercise is enough to release your tension. This is what you will do when you are faced with too much stress and tension:

- Go somewhere quiet and close your eyes.
- Breathe deeply and pay attention to your breathing.
- Breathe in and breathe out.

- Feel how your body feels every time you breathe in and how it feels each time you breathe out.

Continue doing it until you feel lighter. Only open your eyes when you feel relieved and ready to face the present. The exercise will give you a clearer outlook and lighten up your mood. Once you open your eyes, you will feel renewed.

6. Use essential oils

A part of your brain governs your memory and emotions. And near that area is the part responsible for processing scents. This is why scents can induce good emotions and helps calm your mind.

A study published in 2008 proved that intensive care unit nurses who use essential oils found it easier to manage their tension and stress. Dab a little amount on your clothes or skin to use the oils. You can also use a diffuser so that everyone in the room will benefit from it. The most recommended essential oil for combating stress are lavender, ylang-ylang, and peppermint.

In a Nutshell

In this chapter, you have learned more about the roots of stress. Since stress is a big factor why people resort to emotional or binge eating, you have to learn how to combat it.

- Stress is not always bad. Sometimes, it helps you overcome situations you thought you could not do. However, it can also beat the best out of you.
- Aside from emotional eating, frequent stress can also affect your health.
- You can deal with stress using your senses - sight, hearing, smell, touch, taste, and movement.
- This chapter also lists the six effective ways to deal with stress at the moment. It could be as easy as laughing. It can also include meditations and deep breathing.

Let us continue learning about what you can do to defeat stress no matter where you are. In the next chapter, you will learn about stress relief techniques you can follow when it hits you at home or in the office. Let us find out how to make stress-relief habits a part of your lifestyle.

CHAPTER FIVE

Making Stress Relief Part of Your Lifestyle

Whatever the situation, the answer is not in the fridge.

- Anonymous

Never allow yourself to get beaten by stress. We must equip ourselves with knowledge about what to do whenever and wherever it hits.

While learning, ensure you are helping yourself by refraining from eating whenever you're stressed. This is the discipline that you have to master. This is the only way to ensure you'd succeed in the other meditation and hypnosis techniques you need to grasp to lose weight and become healthier.

STRESS RELIEF TECHNIQUES AT HOME

When you are suddenly stressed out while at home, you can use your imagination or any objects that can help relieve the heaviness.

Here are some of the things of can do the moment stress hits you:

- **Think about your childhood**

Use your imagination, close your eyes, and go back to when you were a child. As your mind goes on a trip down memory lane, try to remember the happy memories you had when you were young. Savor these moments until you feel lighter.

- **Think about your parents or elders you've grown up with**

It may not have been clear while you were young, but you may have seen how your parents dealt with stress at the time. You only did not understand back then. If your parents rarely got angry or practiced patience when their kids were rowdy, they may be using stress quick relief techniques. Think about what they used to do to control their temper and anger. Once you have understood and connected the dots, do the same thing to control your raging emotions.

- **Use whatever is available**

Turn off the television and play soothing music instead. Refrain from using technology. Keep your phone away and stay away from any gadgets. Give yourself a break from all these. Music will help calm your nerves. If not, you can also turn off the music and enjoy the silence.

Here are the other techniques you can try to cure stress at home. The next time you feel stressed, just choose among the list what to do and make sure you keep your mind away from food as much as you can:

1. Be comfortable

Live comfortably without minding how you look or what you wear. You are at home so that you can be at your most comfortable. Leave your worries for some time, and be silly. Have fun with your loved ones and forget about your problems in the meantime. You need to experience this feeling when you don't have to prove yourself or compete, even once in a while. This is like a mental break that will recharge and make you feel better.

2. Sleep

The grumpiness may already be caused by the heaviness you feel inside. Your body may be telling you it wants to rest. Take this chance to catch up on your snooze, but make sure you don't overdo it. Oversleeping can make you feel worse. If you're finding it hard to sleep, playing soothing music might help. Make sure the room's temperature is cozy, and you can also try diffusing comforting scents in the area. Most importantly, try to forget about your worries when you go to bed. You wouldn't want to dream about them.

3. Clean

Tidying up your house for 10 to 15 minutes at the start of your day is a form of exercise. Any physical activity can boost your mood and pump up your energy. If you have the time, you may also want to do a general cleaning or a major makeover. Some people feel stressed when they see things in disarray.

Looking at nice surroundings where everything looks clean and in order will help pacify your emotions.

4. Spend time in the kitchen

Many home buddies find the kitchen as their favorite area at home. They find it relaxing when they cook, bake, or get their hands busy with any kitchen work. If you don't like cooking, you may still find comfort in the kitchen by enjoying the aroma. Try smelling the ingredients or the scent coming from the cooked dishes.

5. Make your home a sanctuary

Arrange and design your home to make it a place you will look forward to after a stressful day at work. You can make it pleasing for you by changing the paint's color or covering the walls with wallpapers with calming designs. You can also display images or figurines that make you look happy. Place curtains and diffuse scents each day before you leave. The scents will welcome you when you come home, which will help you feel invigorated.

6. Nurture your relationships

The old cliche, home is where the heart is, is true for many people. Consider yourself lucky if you have your loved ones and a family you come home to. Nurture the relationship by understanding how everyone feels, from the youngest to the oldest family member.

When arguing with your partner, make it a point that your kids do not see or hear you quarrel. However, you need to discuss and resolve the issues before bed. On the other hand, when trying to discipline your kids, refrain from shouting or getting angry as much as possible. Breathe deeply before facing them and try to rationally talk about what they have done.

STRESS RELIEF TECHNIQUES IN THE OFFICE

Most people get stressed in their workplaces. You get stressed by your workmates and bosses, the workload or absence of tasks. No matter how stressful work life may seem, make sure that you don't quit in haste. You have to secure a replacement job or a venture to pursue if you resign. Life will be more stressful if you will lose your income source.

Here are some quick stress-relief you can do in the office to avoid contemplating quitting:

1. Do not overwork yourself

Working beyond your limits will leave you feeling drained and burned out. You will know you are overworked when you become less productive than usual. It can affect your output, and you will become withdrawn and irritable.

Allowing this to continue will lead to the abuse of your physical and mental capacities. You will likely see yourself one day that you no longer find satisfaction with what you're doing.

You have to understand the warning signs and do something about them before worse comes to worst. Here are the factors you need to look out for:

- Trouble concentrating and shorter attention span
- Often getting disinterested and anxious
- Tiredness, even at the start of the day
- Depression
- Having trouble sleeping at night
- Frequent muscle and stomach problems
- Susceptibility to sicknesses

Make sure that you take care of your physical and mental health. Know your limits, and never overwork to the point of getting burned out.

2. Prioritize your health

You are only trying to lose weight and not starve yourself. Your body finds it stressful when it has to work without food in its system. Eat on time and eat right.

3. Learn how to deal with stress depending on what you are doing at work

Remember to breathe deeply if you are in a meeting with people arguing and the ambiance is stressful. Refrain from arguing, and wait until heads are cooled before raising your points. To calm your nerves, you can sip tea or massage the tips of your fingers.

After spending so much time in front of a computer doing repeated tasks, you will feel heavy after a while. To relieve yourself from tension and stress, make it a habit to stand up every hour or so and do simple exercises. Your exercise can be as simple as stretching or knee bends. You can also try using the computer while standing up once in a while. This will help prevent backaches you will likely suffer from sitting for an extended period.

Take the time to walk while talking to someone on the phone. Pace back and forth, but ensure you are not disturbing anyone else in the workplace.

Recharge during lunch or coffee breaks. You can meditate for a few minutes or stroll outside to catch fresh air.

TOP STRATEGIES TO DEAL WITH STRESS WHEREVER YOU ARE

You are on your way to taking full control of your response to stress. This doesn't mean that you won't have slip-ups from time to time. However, it will help to be kind to yourself and accept that you are bound to make mistakes.

You must also make the following techniques part of your lifestyle:

Talking

If you have been keeping everything to yourself - problems, misery, challenges, you are setting yourself up to explode when you least expect it.

Talking is liberating and therapeutic.

You can solve many of your problems, including stress, when you learn to talk and share what you are going through with someone. You need to find a voice and let it be heard. Many things in life will leave you feeling overwhelmed. Talk about it. Find someone who will listen and understand without judgment. When you keep all your emotions inside, it will get to a point when it becomes too much. It might lead to the feeling of getting stuck. Aside from stress, you will likely get depressed or become emotionally frozen.

Life will become harder and more stressful if you hit the wall. So make it a habit to express yourself and share whatever you are going through with someone you trust. While talking will not solve the problem, it will make your feelings lighter.

Talking will clear your mind and help you gain new perspectives.

Keeping your problems to yourself is not healthy. It's hard to reason when you are physically, mentally, and emotionally drained. By sharing your problems with others, they may share their stories with you or those they know who have gone through the same things. This will give you ideas on how to face the problems you have. It feels lighter knowing that other people have gone through the same ordeals. It will also lift your burdens when you have verbalized what you have been keeping inside.

Taking a break

You owe it to yourself to take a break from time to time. Too much work without stopping to recharge can lead to exhaustion, stress, and tension. If you continue like this, do not be surprised to find yourself emotionally, mentally, and physically drained one day. Your body is an engine that stops functioning when it loses fuel. It is also your responsibility to drive the engine without overspeeding and overheating. The engine needs to do a complete stop regularly for a check-up or overhaul.

You need to recharge your body to recover and perform better. It doesn't have to be a once-a-week or once-a-month experience. You can schedule mini-timeouts each day. Each timeout will last for 10 to 15 minutes. For example, you have done a grueling presentation or finished all your tasks for the day. You can do the following to recharge during your mini-timeout:

- Read a chapter of your favorite book.
- Find a quiet space wherever you are and meditate.
- You can bring small exercise tools to the office that you can use during your break, like a dumbbell or a stress ball.
- Power nap.
- Go up and down the stairs for several minutes.

Making it a habit

After learning all the effective strategies for dealing with stress, you must keep doing what works for you. It will also help to try other things that did not work initially. This way, you won't get easily bored with how you deal with stress. No matter what you do, keep your focus on your goals. You want to lose weight. You can only do that if you will keep your mind off food every time you are faced with a stressful situation.

To make the stress relief techniques part of your lifestyle, you must do them as often as possible or whenever needed. You can begin with the following stress-busting tips you can integrate into your everyday life:

1. Keep healthy snacks within reach

You never know when stress and real hunger will hit you at the same time. When your tummy is already grumbling, not because you're stressed but because you are really hungry, you've got to eat. This is no time for deep breathing or strolling outside. You need food.

But what if it happens while you are in the office and it is still not your break time? To ease your hunger at times like this, it is best when you can easily reach something you can munch that will make you forget about the hunger, even for a few minutes or some hours.

While bidding your time and trying to relieve hunger, you can have a piece of dark chocolate. You may also want to keep a handful of healthy nuts you can munch on. Have plenty of water and fruit juices within reach as well.

2. Get organized

We tend to forget many things as we grow older. This can lead to stress, especially when we need to remember something badly. We can make it easier by creating a list. Before sleeping at night, list down all the things you need to accomplish the next day. If you'd be leaving the house, list all things you need to bring. Check the list upon waking up and prepare everything. Once in your workplace, check the list and ensure you accomplish all tasks you've written on it.

3. Make the stress relief strategies part of your routine

If you are doing yoga, meditation, or hypnosis, perform them at the start of each day. Whenever you have a chance to walk, do it, and take the chance to breathe fresh air. You also have to practice deep breathing every hour or two.

4. Keep your hands clean

Your immune system becomes low when you're stressed and pressured. Low immunity makes you susceptible to viruses and germs. The simple act of washing your hands can help in protecting your immunity. You can do it whenever you have a chance or while taking a break.

5. Listen to music

Make it a habit to find comfort in music. When in the workplace, listen to it with your earphones on. This way, you won't cause a distraction to other people working in the area.

6. Swimming

If you have a pool at home, swimming at the start of the day or before sleeping at night can help lower stress levels.

7. Self-appreciation

Always remind yourself that you are doing something right. Give yourself a pat on the back for every job well done. Tell yourself that you are doing good, so you don't need to worry.

8. Self-talk or journaling

You can look in the mirror and talk to yourself whenever you are alone. Tell yourself everything you want to say - good or bad. Rant and do not edit yourself. You can also shower yourself with praises if that's what you are in the mood for. If you are too self-conscious to do it, you can opt to write all that you have to say to yourself in your journal.

9. Schedule a full body massage at least once a month

The massage and touch therapy feel nurturing and comforting. Having a full-body massage can lighten up your burden.

We'll have more about reflexology in the coming chapters. This is also a good massage technique that focuses on points or areas in the body that corresponds to one's chakras or ailing body parts. This is easier to learn, and you can do it on your own or with your loved one.

10. Always be positive and thankful

No matter your problem, always find reasons to smile and be happier. Say thanks for everything you are grateful for at the end of each day.

With continued practice, you will learn how to integrate stress-relief techniques into your everyday life. The techniques will eventually feel more natural as you do them more often. The best thing about it is that you are developing proper ways to deal with your stress by understanding the causes. This will make it easier for you to deal with your weight loss journey.

In a Nutshell

This chapter is about making stress relief a daily habit.

- Think about the good memories you can hold on to and reflect on whenever you feel burdened with stress. By learning how to deal with it, you will have more success in preventing binge eating.
- Life will be lighter, and you will become healthier once you've learned to deal with stress efficiently. You can

practice the steps at home, in the office, or wherever stress hits you.

- From now on, you will make the stress-relief habits part of your lifestyle. Be grateful, thankful, and always positive no matter what life brings your way.

CHAPTER SIX

Taking Actions Towards a Healthier You

Respect yourself enough to walk away from anything that no longer serves you, grows you, or makes you happy.

- Robert Tew

The previous chapters taught you about dealing with the inner struggles that make you reach out to food. You already know why it is hard to resist emotional eating when emotionally unstable.

It's time to take action and do something about the problem.

You are on your way. You've already dealt with it in your mind and emotions. You are now going to do something about your weight issues through actions.

This chapter will make you realize that you have made the right choice - to become healthier without taking pills, following fad diets, or to starve yourself. You have broken free from the cycle of emotional eating and have developed a healthier relationship with food.

Let's bring awareness to how you can make healthy choices by learning about nutrition and healthy eating.

RESPECT YOUR BODY'S BALANCED STATE

Your body has a naturally balanced state, and that is what you have to respect. To sustain it, you must eat a wide range of food items from different food groups. You don't have to restrict yourself by following a complicated diet that will destroy the balance. Eating right will make it easier to sustain yourself with the daily recommended amounts of minerals, vitamins, and macronutrients (protein, carbohydrates, and fats).

Healthy eating is simple. You only have to keep things simple. Things get tricky when you overcomplicate them. According to the American USDA and the British FSA, a healthy diet is high in starchy whole grains (1/3 of your intake) and fruits and vegetables (1/3 of your intake). The rest of the proportion is split between dairy foods and protein.

Here's what you need to remember. The food we eat is categorized into five major food groups - dairy or milk products, non-dairy protein, starchy foods and grains, fruits, and vegetables.

Here are the three crucial things you have to remember to eat simply:

1. In consuming food, it is best to eat them without sugars, fats, added salt, and processing elements, such as preservatives, flavoring, and artificial sweeteners. It is healthier to eat food in its most dense state.
2. Not all foods that belong to the same food groups are equal.
3. Follow the right proportions and make it easier by thinking in thirds: 1/3 dairy and protein, 1/3 grains and starch, and 1/3 fruits and vegetables.

Many fad diets sell their ideas by promoting more or less consumption of protein, carbs, or fats. These three comprise the macronutrients in your diet. Without them or having too little or any of the three will result in medical issues and severe malnutrition.

Let's learn more about protein, carbohydrates, and fats and why they are essential in a healthy diet:

Protein

Your body needs protein to build tissue and cells your body requires to function well. Without enough protein, your body will turn to the protein found in your tissues and muscles to digest.

On the other hand, your kidney will suffer when you consume too much protein, especially when most of it comes from meat containing high levels of saturated fat. Diets recommending no or low carbs to focus mainly on protein is not healthy either. It will make you weak. The best sources of protein include pulses, seeds, nuts, soya beans, poultry, lean meat, and eggs. You can also get it from red meat, but it is not advisable to consume it often since it may contain high amounts of saturated fat.

Carbohydrates

They are your body's main energy source. Restricting yourself of carbs will force your system to use protein for energy. This is done by processing the proteins in the muscles. Allowing this to continue can cause heart ailments and death.

Sufficient carbs help maintain healthy sugar levels that decrease cravings and boost energy.

The classification of carbs regarding how they are processed and utilized by the body is called the Glycaemic Index (GI). Foods containing high GI are absorbed by the body faster. As a result, you will experience a sudden surge of energy but also a fast decline in your blood sugar shortly after. On the other hand, low GI foods minimize slumps and spikes since they give your body more consistent blood sugar levels. They also make you feel full for a longer time, whereas high GI foods have the opposite effect.

How would you know the GI content of the food you buy? You will usually find the GI rating in the food packaging if you buy them in supermarkets. Some samples of low GI foods are oranges, apples, sweet potato, wheat pasta, pulses, oats, and new potatoes. It is recommended to consume low GI food in each meal to make it easier to sustain healthy blood sugar levels. Goods with a high GI, which you have to consume minimally, include sweets, biscuits, cakes, chips, crackers, whole meal bread, and white bread.

Fats

Your body needs fats and oils for many processes, including hormone formation, brain and nerve functions, and cell membrane formation. Fat also helps your system process the A, E, D, and K vitamins, which are crucial for healthy blood, bones, eyesight, hair, and skin.

However, not all fats have the same effects. You have to stay away from food sources containing high amounts of saturated fat. They include animal products and meat. Trans-fats are also unhealthy and are found in processed food, including biscuits, cookies, cakes, and pastries.

The healthy fats you need to constantly supply your body with are seed oils, plant and nut oils, fish oils, omega 3, and omega 6.

PROPER EATING HABITS TO LOSE WEIGHT AND MAINTAIN A GOOD FIGURE

Here are the steps you need to remember regarding eating habits to make it easier to focus on your wellness goals:

1. Eat less than your Resting Metabolic Rate

Resting Metabolic Rate is also referred to as BMR or Basal Metabolic Rate. It pertains to the number of calories your body burns while resting. These calories are essential for the body's basic functions, such as breathing and circulation.

Knowing your BMR makes it easy to calculate the number of calories you need to burn to lose weight. It doesn't mean that you have to spend too much of your time counting the calories. After practicing it for a week or two, you will already have an idea. You only have to pattern your calorie consumption in your previous intake. Our daily caloric intake depends on gender, age, height (inches), and weight (pounds).

2. Drink plenty of water

Drinking plenty of water can boost your metabolism and suppress your appetite. The old rule of eight to ten glasses daily is still the best to follow up to this day. Drinking plenty of water will lower your calorie consumption. Drink water before each meal or snack. Aside from making you feel full faster, the water will also aid digestion by making it easier to break down. This way, the nutrients will be absorbed by your body faster.

Another method you can try is a detox water diet. But make sure that you only do it for a short duration that won't exceed one week. When done longer than a week, your body will lack the essential nutrients required to perform and get energized. This is done by infusing fresh veggies and fruits in clean water. You can add flavors like mint leaves, melons, citrus fruits, herbs, and cucumbers.

Cut the fruits or veggies you will use, soak in water and leave in the fridge for an hour or two before drinking. You can choose to use only one flavor or mix two or more. The infused water will last for three days when refrigerated and a day when left at room temperature.

3. Eat clean, unprocessed foods

It is possible to lose up to three pounds or more in a week when you adapt to a clean eating lifestyle. This means that you will eat foods that are good for you. These include carbohydrates, whole grains, vegetables, fruits, healthy fats, and lean protein. Eat enough portion sizes six times a day. This is better instead of eating major meals three times a day. You won't get hungry in between meals by dividing the meals into smaller portions and eating them throughout the day.

4. Limit your sugar intake

If you have become too used to consuming too much sugar, you may find it hard to cut down your consumption at once. You can start slow to give your body enough time to adjust to the changes. It is estimated that around 16% of the calories in an average American diet are composed of added sugar. You can only imagine how much weight you'd lose if you could limit your sugar intake.

This is not easy. Sugar has addicting properties that make it hard to cut down on it. You don't have to eliminate your favorite desserts into your diet. Allow yourself to indulge once in a while but make sure to avoid too much consumption. Low sugar intake will help you lose weight and make you less vulnerable to sicknesses, such as heart disease, cancer, and diabetes.

ESSENTIAL STEPS TO HEALTHY EATING

Post this list in your fridge or any space where you will often see it. This way, you will be reminded constantly of the important factors that will help you in shedding off the unwanted pounds fast:

- Listen to your hunger. Eat only when you are hungry and not when you think you should eat. Stop eating once you are full.
- Do not use the microwave in cooking or heating foods. This appliance destroys the nutrients in your food. Having a microwave also makes it tempting to eat ready meals often. These meals are highly processed, have low nutrients, and are loaded with salt, sugar, and fat.
- Eat your foods right. As much as possible, eat fruits and vegetables raw. They are more nutritious in their natural state.
- Your metabolism slows down at night because your system is getting ready to sleep, so it conserves energy.

Make sure that you avoid munching on anything when it's already late.

- Eat breakfast. It is the meal that pumps up your metabolism after it rested while you were sleeping. This meal will give you the energy to last up to the next meal of the day.
- Drink plenty of water. It cleanses your system and aids digestion.
- Consume protein sources that do not contain saturated fat.
- Include low GI carbs in your every meal.
- The main components of your meals must be starchy foods and vegetables.
- If you have access to organic foods, go organic whenever possible.
- Avoid consuming processed foods since they contain little to no nutrients at all.
- Limit your intake of foods with preservatives, flavorings, bad fats, sugar, and added salt.
- All food groups are crucial to health. Respect the naturally balanced state of your body.

HOW TO DEAL WITH YOUR CRAVINGS?

Cravings hit when you least expect them, even when you are full. No matter how intent you are on losing weight, you will experience occasional cravings that would be hard to resist. Cravings happen when your mind says you want it even though your body says no. To deal with the sudden cravings and sustain your nutrition goals, you must convince your mind that you don't want to eat.

Meditation Time

Here's what you can do to banish the sudden cravings:

Go to your quiet spot and be in your most comfortable position.

Focus on the food you often crave, but you would be okay not to eat ever again.

Close your eyes. Focus on the food you've chosen. Imagine how it looks and feels when touched. Imagine the texture of this food once you've placed it in your mouth. When you chew it, imagine how it feels. When you swallow, imagine the sensation it brings. Visualize that you are eating a big chunk of this food while experiencing all the sensations it brings.

Open your eyes. Think of something you will never dare eat, like a live bug, dirt on the ground, or smelly trash. It can also be food that you find disgusting. Close your eyes. Imagine that thing that you would not want to eat. Visualize it on a plate in front of you. Focus on its smell, texture, and appearance.

While keeping your eyes closed, place the food you're craving for to the disgusting food on your plate. Mix them. Visualize the tastes, textures, and smells getting combined. Imagine a foul smell coming from what's in front of you. Imagine it coming nearer, and you can almost taste it.

Chew. Imagine that you are eating the disgusting combination. Imagine the sensations and try hard to swallow them. Imagine how it feels while trying to swallow, even if you gag or puke.

Open your eyes. Remind yourself that each time you crave the food you thought of initially, remember the sensations you've had after mixing it with the disgusting element.

Many recommend a faster way to stop cravings without meditating - brushing your teeth. The instant a craving hits you, go to the bathroom and have your teeth cleaned. Seeing how clean your teeth are and how minty your breath smells will stop the craving.

Focused Thinking to Make Healthier Choices

Make a list of suggestions you will remind yourself when choosing snacks, preparing home meals, eating out, and shopping. You can make or add your own, but here are some samples:

"I love preparing food for myself and loved ones whenever I'm home. I make sure to combine textures, colors, aromas, and flavors. I use healthy ingredients and prepare foods in ways that I will maximize the nutrients they contain."

"I always check the menu when eating out and make healthy choices. I go for quality nutrient-dense meals loaded with natural flavors."

"I skip the aisle when doing grocery shopping. I am aware that it's where the processed foods, sugary drinks, crisps, and biscuits are. This is my way of respecting the naturally balanced state of my body and my commitment to my goal of getting fitter."

"When I shop for food, I always include vegetables and fruits. I enjoy these nutritious foods and use them in preparing healthy and delicious meals."

In a Nutshell

This chapter starts teaching you how to take action after learning how to control emotional eating by dealing with the causes.

- Respect your body's naturally balanced state by eating a wide range of foods that belong to the different food groups.
- Supply your body with the five major food groups to keep it healthy - dairy or milk products, non-dairy

protein, starchy foods and grains, fruits, and vegetables.

- You have to consume enough protein, carbohydrates, and fats.
- You can resist cravings through meditation or by keeping your teeth clean.
- Ultimately, it is your responsibility to your body and your loved ones to make healthier choices always.

Before we focus on the physical aspect of becoming healthier, let's learn more about the other hypnosis techniques that can help you lose weight. In the next chapter, I'll discuss hypnosis ideas that are easy to follow and effective in helping you achieve your fitness goals.

CHAPTER SEVEN

More about Hypnosis and Weight Loss

> *It's okay to struggle, but it's not okay to give up on*
> *yourself or your dreams.*
> *- Gabe Grunewald*

Hypnosis is a method that aims to reach the unconscious mind. It involves many techniques, but these strategies aim to induce a positive change.

Different persons may require to undergo varying hypnosis techniques. This is because each individual is unique. The therapist will find the most suitable approach to which you will likely respond.

Here are the hypnosis techniques typically used in weight loss:

- Reframing
- Mind disassociation
- Changing perspectives
- Awareness of needs
- Gastric band hypnosis

We will start with these four before going into the other techniques and alternative methods to deal with your weight issues.

HYPNOSIS TECHNIQUE TO LOSE WEIGHT - REFRAMING

Reframing makes it possible for a person to hold their stand. They will not easily fall into the trap of resigning themselves to bad habits because they have convinced themselves that it is possible to change. The technique is all about reframing the subconscious. By doing so, you start defeating the cliches, including "I am too tired to exercise," "I need to eat junk food," or "I will no longer get fit. I only have to live with it."

With this technique, you won't easily get defeated by such thoughts. You will tell a new story instead of repeating the cliches, bad thoughts, or habits. With reframing, you will change - I am "bad habit," to I was challenged by "bad habit." You will think about the bad habit as a challenge you need to overcome instead of resigning and accepting defeat early on.

What is Reframing?

Whatever thoughts you often have, you will become that person. If you think negatively too often, you tend to become a negative person without intending to. If this continues, it will impact your life and reduce its quality. Being too negative all the time will limit how you enjoy life. It will make you less confident and less happy.

You have to think this way - you were not born a negative person; no one is. This is a behavior people learn. We live according to what we've learned. And if we have trained our thoughts to become consistently negative, that's what we become; that's the part we pursue to play.

However, hypnosis can help you stop these negative thoughts by replacing and changing them. Everything begins with your thoughts, which control your feelings that, in turn, control your actions, which tell you how to behave. This is the process that goes by to your thoughts. You justify everything in your mind.

So if your mind says you can't lose weight, your feelings will get sad, which will prompt you to reach your comfort foods. Until it becomes a behavior - you reach for food whenever you're sad. Your mind will process the cycle and justify everything by saying, "It's okay. At least this makes you feel good."

But you do really feel good? How could you when you are no longer happy with what the excess food is doing to your body? It is not happiness when you get satisfaction only when you eat but regret it afterward. It is not happiness when you shy away from meeting people because you are ashamed of how big you have gotten, or you no longer feel confident with your own body.

Changing your thinking will change your life. You can start by changing your negative thoughts into positive ones.

Where does negative thinking come from? Think about this. When you were born, you came out full of positive thoughts. Children seem to have an answer for everything. For example, if people don't have money, they go to a bank because they will get money there. When adults complain of rains, many children say that rains help flowers bloom.

This is the kind of positive thinking that you have to emanate. You have to think like a child. Of course, in a sensible way, since you now understand that you can't simply go to the bank to get money if you don't have a saving account, or that too much rain may also cause the plants to get destroyed. But instead of pondering on the negative, you take action. You start saving up early in life. You put the plants that might get flooded by the rains inside your home.

You don't overthink how fat you already are. You decide to take action, tell yourself you can do this, and take the necessary steps to lose the extra pounds.

If children are idealistic and always see the brighter side of things, where do they learn the negativity? Sadly, adults teach them to be negative. You will see the difference in children being exposed to adults' negativity. They will start thinking negatively in advance of a situation.

They would go like, "We'll never make it on time," "There will be too many people at the mall, you won't find any parking space," or "It's impossible to find the toy I like at this store."

The fact is that a negative person thinks negative thoughts and makes them real. Sadly, it is rooted in the people that raised us. If you grew up with adults always thinking that negative things will happen before even trying.

There's a difference between a parent telling their kids not to climb a tree because they're going to fall and parents telling their kids to be careful and watch their steps and where they place their hands as they climb the tree. A child who was told she was going to fall will likely fall.

Most parents might have the best intention for their kids, but by becoming too negative, you are teaching your kids not to take risks. This is when the transition happens of people learning to be negative. They start thinking small. They stick to what is familiar because it makes them feel safe.

But your brain can be trained. You can teach yourself to break free from all the effects of too much negativity.

You can begin by stopping saying the word "but." For example, you told yourself that you would start losing weight. This is a positive thought. Then you will add - but I can't stop eating ice cream because it makes me feel happy.

Once you utter the word "but," you return to what's familiar. You are disregarding your first conviction of losing weight because you have thought about how food makes you feel after saying the word "but."

Other people would say that they can't wake up early to do exercises. They can't eat healthy foods because they are not delicious. These thoughts mean that you are sticking with what's familiar. There are no weight loss programs that you will find easy to try or think you could pursue if you will not push yourself beyond what's familiar.

Reframing focuses on making positive thoughts familiar and negative thoughts unfamiliar. This way, it will be easier for you to embrace positivity while disregarding your negative thoughts.

Reframing Your Thoughts to Lose Weight

Let's try this one out. First, you must find a quiet spot and sit in a comfortable chair. Sit like you're a free person. Sit as comfortably as you can without crossing your legs or arms. If you can open your arms and legs, much better.

Focus, stop fiddling and get ready to understand. Unlike popular beliefs, hypnosis is not scary. This won't make you fall asleep. In fact, this will wake your senses with all the amazing possibilities of who you are and what you can achieve when you choose to think positively.

Thinking positive is a choice. So before starting, you have to choose to become a positive person.

Let's begin.

1. Look up like how your eyes would stare into nothingness when you're preparing to sleep. Keep your lids down and your eyeballs up as if you're looking into the top of your forehead.

2. Keep your feet apart and make sure your hands are not touching. Look up as high as you can.

3. Breathe in and breathe out. Keep your eyeballs up as you continue breathing in and breathing out for a few seconds.

4. Slowly drop your chin as if you're looking down a flight of stairs with about ten steps.

5. As you look down, you can see your feet and feel the looking down sensation. As your feet move at step ten, feel every nerve, every muscle turns loose. Go deeper.

6. Take your feet to step nine. Now calmly and gently move on to a deeper level.

7. Take step eight. Now you must feel your feet connecting to every step and go deeper.

8. Take step seven. Hear your feet as they touch every step as you go even deeper.

9. Take step six. Look at your feet and hear the sounds they make. Feel your feet connected to each step you make. Allow yourself to go deeper until you open a profound awareness of who you are.

10. Take step five. Go deeper with every sound you hear - your own heartbeat and your own breathing. Go even deeper.

11. As you take step four, gently and beautifully make yourself drift to the wonderful state of healing hypnosis.

12. Take step three as you continue getting deeper.

13. Take step two and feel each nerve, each muscle turns loose, and go deeper.

14. Continue going deeper and sink deeper as you take step one. Listen with your subconscious mind as you go deeper.

15. As you go deeper, let your mind remind you of being a newborn baby with people looking at you, curious about how you are. This baby felt excited about everything and was born with endless possibilities. Babies feel happy with the simplest of things and can spend hours looking at the same things.

If you have forgotten how it was like to be a baby, start reactivating and recreating the ability you were born with to be positive.

You can make changes with yourself twice each day - with how you think and how you act and react. Right now, you have chosen to be positive. After doing the steps above, you have made the decision to be positive.

From now on, start each day by saying, "I'm choosing to be positive and feel great about it." Start now, and say it out loud.

As you do this every day, you are sending a message to your mind that you want to be positive, and you choose it because being positive is a choice. Tell yourself, "I choose to be positive, and I love it."

As you go deeper and as your mind hears these things, it will start manifesting the thoughts. It will make your mind act upon what it hears. It acts upon the words you say.

So, say it again:

"I'm choosing to be positive and feel great about it. Being positive is who I am, and who I am is positive."

As you say the words, your mind thinks it. And as the process continues, you will start to become a walking, living, talking, powerful example of a positive being.

How do you apply positive thinking to your goal of losing weight?

The next time you wake up, you will decide to start doing something about your weight. Tell yourself that you can do it, that it is something you can achieve. Then act on it. Begin your day by exercising. And as the day goes by, choose the food and the amount you take to help you with your goal of losing weight.

You will feel freer through the days as you begin seeing the results of your actions. The idea here is to always think about how to make any thought positive.

To make positive thinking a habit, you have to learn how to flip over negative thoughts.

If your old negative thoughts would say - "Exercise will only tire me out." Flip it, and think, "Exercise will boost my energy."

Say "I can do it" instead of "I can't do it."

And each day, these positive thoughts will sink in deeper into your skin and into your thoughts. These words will nourish you each day until you realize that how you see the world depends on the words you say to yourself and the pictures you put into your head.

With reframing hypnosis, you make positive words and pictures because you choose to be positive.

So every day, you will choose to do two positive things. Choose positive words and put positive images in your head. It all boils down to the truth that the only thing you can control is your thoughts.

HYPNOSIS TECHNIQUE TO LOSE WEIGHT - MIND DISASSOCIATION

A hypnotherapist uses this to change the perspective of a patient. A person typically associates themselves with their thoughts. They think their thoughts define them and can't control their feelings over whatever goes inside their minds.

This technique is used to separate the person from their thoughts. The concept of Mind Disassociation is to disassociate one's physical body and thoughts from what or who they are as a person. This allows them to become an outsider observing their thoughts, enabling them to understand and better control their thoughts instead of allowing them to dictate their actions.

What is Mind Disassociation?

In hypnosis, disassociation uses non-linear inductions. It's the very opposite of authoritative inductions we're familiar with in hypnosis or telling what the patient needs to do.

Disassociation allows the hypnotherapist to become more permissive, unpredictable, and non-linear when dealing with patients. This technique makes it more difficult for patients to predict what will happen next, catching them off guard and unable to fight against the induction.

Disassociation happens when one or more mental tasks lose their connection, making the consciousness unable to access a particular element in mind. Some circumstances, such as trauma, can cause disassociation. But hypnotherapists can influence disassociation to make it becomes therapeutic. Through this type of hypnosis, you will be induced to experience changes in perceptions, sensations, thoughts, and behavior by the power of suggestion.

Aside from weight loss, hypnosis can be used alone or in combination with other treatment methods to deal with the symptoms of certain conditions, including phobias, pain, anxiety, depression, and more.

It is said that hypnosis started in ancient Egypt and Greece. Jame Brais, a pioneer in the field, mastered how to make people fix their attention on an object and then put them into a trance once done. This has paved the way for the popular depiction of hypnosis in media, showing the use of swinging watches to put people in a trance.

Dissociation as a Defense Mechanism

Dissociation is said to be something that everybody does. It is an adaptive defense that people with trauma or high-stress use as a response, especially when the disconnect has something to do with one's surroundings, oneself, and memory loss. It is naturally ingrained in a person's system to survive or help you cope with what could be an overwhelming or defeating feeling of going through too much stress (Steinberg and Schnall, 2001).

Guided Meditation for Disassociation

If you want to heal using disassociation, you have to accept that the healing must begin with you. This guided meditation can help you heal in whatever you are going through, not just about weight loss or keeping your shape. You can focus on the roots of the problem - what brought you here?

Why do you need this guided meditation now? What is bothering you?

The fact that you are here now and you are continuing to read this entry means that you want to get past something. You are suffering from an emotional or mental dilemma that you find hard to get past.

After accepting that you need help, be prepared to go through this guided meditation for dissociation. Go somewhere quiet and where you cannot be disturbed for the next 15 minutes or so. Do not bring anything that may disturb you, like your pet or phone. Go to a spot where you will feel relaxed and at peace.

You can sit or lay down, whatever position you'd feel most comfortable.

Let's begin.

Breathe deeply, and focus on your breath. Breath in through the nose and breath out through your mouth.

Continue breathing in and out as you allow your body to feel more relaxed. As you do, your breathing will become calmer and more even.

Focus on your breathing as you allow everything you hear in the room to fade slowly; allow all that you hear outside of the room to fade. Start shifting your focus inward.

Place one hand on your abdomen and one hand on your heart. Feel the sensations underneath your hands as you gently breathe in through your nose until the air reaches your abdomen and breathe out through your mouth. Feel as your hands rise and fall with each breath.

In your mind, talk to yourself and say, "I am breathing. This is my breath."

Now focus on the hand on top of your chest, and feel your heartbeat. In your mind, talk to yourself and say, "This pulse is why I am alive. It supplies fresh oxygenated blood all over my body. This is my heartbeat. I am alive."

Focus on the sensations you feel throughout your body. If you have any lingering thoughts, focus on them. Now, allow your mind and body to be still.

Whenever you find your mind wandering, bring your focus on your breath by breathing in through your nose and out through your mouth.

Now move your attention to your feet down to the soles. Feel how they are relaxed with whatever your position is. Hold on to the feeling, and bring it up to your knees, thighs, hips, and abdomen. Feel the rise and fall of your abs as you continue breathing in and breathing out.

Now, focus on your hands, each of your fingers, and then on your palms. Keep the focus as you bring it to your chest underneath your hand and feel your heart beating.

Move your awareness up to your throat and swallow. Feel your neck as you do.

Go higher, and bring your focus to your face. Breathe in and out through the nose and feel the air as you do.

Bring your awareness to the top of your head. Focus on the area where the scalp meets the air. Imbibe the feeling. Focus on the area, and then imagine a bright white light entering into it. Imagine the light entering your body. Feel it. Feel the light fill your entire body as you bring your awareness with it. Open yourself and let the light fill you.

Gradually, bring your mind back to your breathing.

Breath in through your nose. Breath out through your mouth. Continue breathing deeply to get your body more relaxed and calm.

What you just did is disassociation. It's a practice of detaching from your physical body, which you can do whenever you are stressed or undergoing certain traumas.

You may not be successful on your first try at doing this guided meditation at first. But it will become easier as you do it more often. The exercise has short-term benefits. You will begin the difference after you've done it.

However, when you do this more often, you will start dissociating without even realizing it.

What does this do? The practice will reconnect you to your physical form while staying connected and present.

It is something that you can do every day. Or you can also subject yourself to this meditation at times when you feel detached.

This is the best gift you can give to yourself - being one and connecting with who you are, with every part of your being. This is beneficial for your body and mind.

HYPNOSIS TECHNIQUE TO LOSE WEIGHT - CHANGING PERSPECTIVES

A person's subconscious mind can be border to being unimaginative. It happens when you believe in something and won't let anything dissuade you from doing so. You cling to one option, attitude, or perspective, with your mind closed that there are alternatives.

For example, if you grew up seeing people around you cope with their emotional battles by bingeing on sweets or chocolates, especially when they are sad, nervous, or stressed, you'd grow up thinking that it is the only way to deal with the negative emotions. When it happens to be you going through similar situations, you no longer think about what else to do or how things can be better; you choose to follow what you know, and that is by overeating sweets and chocolates.

This kind of hypnosis will tap into your subconscious and introduce an alternative reality. It will tell your subconscious that there are other options - that you can escape reality for a while by reading, or you can engage in physical activities, such as exercise, that release the happy hormones or endorphins into your system.

What is Changing Perspectives?

This hypnosis technique will help you see a new point of view to gather new perspectives from whatever is dragging you down. It doesn't only have to be about your weight, but if it is your major concern at the moment, then you can focus on that.

However, you can use this hypnosis technique to veer away from your reality for some minutes. It will help you unburden the load. It will make you feel lighter in the end.

By seeing things from a new perspective, even for some minutes or so, you will have a clearer mind. So when you go back to your reality, you can have renewed hope and energy to take action on whatever has been causing you sleepless nights and gloomy days.

It's not only you. Many people are going through whatever you are feeling at the moment. This is part of life, which can be pretty complicated. It is only that people respond to the challenges and the complications differently.

The challenge here is to realize that each of us sees the world only through our eyes, our own perspectives. We hear the world through our own ears.

No matter how much you try to understand the world from another person's point of view, it will never be factual but only an approximation. We can never truly see from someone else's point of view because we can never be on their minds.

But this doesn't mean that you can't try.

Each of us has our own pain, pleasures, and experiences, the good and the bad times. We all have an imagination. We can try to do our best to see things from a new perspective that is not ours.

Are you willing to try?

If the answer is yes, go to a quiet spot where you will not be bothered for five minutes or so. Relax and close your eyes.

With your eyes closed, focus on becoming aware of your own perspective. Feel how your body is feeling. Focus on how your heart beats and how you are breathing.

Be aware of your appearance, body frame, and facial features. Notice your body's reaction to what you are currently doing. Are your lips smiling or frowning?

The more aware you become, the more you will realize that this is the vessel you use to look into the world. You only look through your eyes, taste with your tongue, hear with your ears. You only experience the world all the time through your body.

There is nothing wrong with that. However, there will come a time when you realize that it limits you and what you see. The fact is that your actions do not always appear to others as how you see them through your eyes.

This is where you can play with your mind and use your imagination.

The more you focus on your body, the more you will become aware of it, and the more you can let it go.

For now, focus on the thought that your body no longer matters just for this moment.

Be comfortable as much as you can, and focus on this hypnosis because, for now, this is only what matters.

Listen to the words, for this is the only thing your body has to do, while the rest can take care of it on their own.

Breathe deeply, and imagine all pieces falling into place as you keep on listening.

Now let's focus on your mind, which is an amazingly powerful place. Your mind fuels your fantasies. It directs your dreams. Your mind can allow you to imagine the world or even beyond in a blink of an eye. Your mind creates simple symphonies and complex patterns in and out of your thoughts.

Allow your mind to take you back and forth between consciousness and your unconscious. As the words drift in and out of your consciousness, your mind will help you listen. It will find ways to listen. As it happens, you will become more aware of your own perspective, and the more you can move forward.

All the dreams you dream of are yours. Your mind creates these dreams by listening to the outside world. As your imagination responds to sensations, sounds, and sights, a filter always exists.

This filter may be necessary, but sometimes, you can try letting go of that filter. As you learn how to let go of your own perspective, the more your mind becomes open to new perspectives.

The world does not have absolute truths. You have a lot of perspectives you can choose to see things from. Your life is only one of the billions, meaning that your perspective is also only one of the billions.

Keep trying to step out of your mind, outside your body, and outside your own perspective. The more you do, the more profound and beautiful your understanding of others and yourself become.

When you try your best to understand something or someone from a different perspective, the more you understand the position. This will make you feel better.

The more you understand why someone else does what they did, the more forgiving you become.

The most beautiful thing to do for your mind as you go through this process is letting things go.

The more peaceful your mind is, the easier it becomes to have and accept a new perspective.

It feels good to let go of your point of view, even for a while, as you allow other people's truths to become your truth. The more you allow yourself to see things from other's point of view, the easier it becomes to resolve conflicts and misunderstandings. You will have more fun talking to other people and hearing their words so that you can understand them deeply.

The more you practice letting go of your own perspective while allowing your mind to remain calm and at peace, the more rewarding the process becomes, even though you are not doing this for the reward.

You are doing this because it makes you better. It allows you to embrace people's differences. It helps you grow.

This makes it easier for you to enjoy life to the fullest.

Hopefully, this practice will train your mind to open itself to a new perspective every day,

HYPNOSIS TECHNIQUE TO LOSE WEIGHT - AWARENESS OF NEEDS

This hypnosis technique taps into your subconscious and reminds it to be constantly vigilant. It talks to the subconscious to help it understand the reaction or reasons. It makes you ask questions instead of accepting everything because it has always been like that.

For example, hypnosis creates a subconscious alert when you are craving comfort food because you are feeling down and want to feel better. It makes you stop and think before getting the food or putting it into your mouth.

This hypnosis technique makes you ask - Is this really what I need? Am I hungry to eat? How can this make me happy? Do I really want to eat this, or am I only stressed?

Once you have identified the reasons for your cravings, you begin accepting that there are alternatives, that you can still feel better even without eating the food in front of you, and that you don't need to eat. It makes you seek better alternatives to deal with whatever you are going through.

In hypnosis, some of the methods done as alternatives to the common ways most people deal with their emotional battles include the following:

- Storytelling
- Memory substitution
- Indirect and direct suggestions
- Parts therapy
- Regression
- Visualization
- Learning ways to forget

THE GASTRIC BAND HYPNOSIS

Despite the previously mentioned hypnosis techniques being effective, there is one specifically designed for weight loss and maintaining your shape while keeping off the unwanted fats. It's called the gastric band hypnosis or Hypno band.

It has a similar concept to gastric bypass surgery. This operation makes the digestive system shorter and the stomach smaller. This way, most of the food you ingest goes out directly to defecation without allowing the calories to get absorbed by the body and turn them into fat.

Using hypnosis for weight loss is effective for people who have tried everything to shed off the excess pounds but keep on coming back to unhealthy habits. They are induced to have a healthier outlook toward food. They are made to understand that they need to eat when hungry and not when they are sad, stressed, or fearful.

Let's admit that it is easy to succumb to unhealthy eating. This is why we keep foods in the fridge that we can easily get "just in case." Check your fridge. Do you have a stock of your favorite chocolates, ice cream, cake, and other foods we don't need to have constantly?

If yes, how often do you eat them? If you eat them more often than usual or instantly reach out to these comfort foods whenever you feel off, you have to accept that you have developed an unhealthy relationship with them.

Gastric band hypnosis is hypnotherapy that will induce your subconscious to convince it that you have a smaller stomach. It will make your mind believe that you have undergone gastric bypass surgery (even if you did not) to make you think and eat like someone who had undergone surgery.

The hypnotherapist will guide your subconscious into thinking that a surgeon has operated on your stomach. They tied a band around your stomach to make it smaller. As a result, no matter how small the portions of the food you eat, you tend to feel full at a faster rate.

The catch here is that no actual surgery happened. It's all in the mind. The hypnotherapist only allows you to think differently from how you thought before. It guides your mind to convince you that you are full whenever you tend to reach for food. The Hypno band makes you think you have a smaller stomach, so you can't overeat because it may cause the stomach to rupture.

The gastric band hypnosis is a radical hypnotic surgery technique created to help reprogram your subconscious mind. This aims to help you lose weight fast, with your band becoming tighter after each session.

The indications that it is working are feeling fuller fast and a decrease in your appetite.

It is recommended to do this for 30 days to make this work. Listen to it while lying to experience a complete subconscious reprogramming. After 30 days or less of undergoing the session, you will feel more clamor to reach for liquid than solid foods.

Give in to the clamor, especially at the start of your day. This clamor will begin after each session. You can take in gentle liquids, such as raw juices and smoothies. It's also important to consume at least three liters of water during the day. Depending on the weather, you may also eat soups or ice lollipops.

However, your body may respond differently each day. You may only want water and juices the first day but would crave soups the next day.

Additionally, day by day, you will be able to gauge the right quantity of meals suited for your body - just right, nothing too much. Smaller and lighter meals will be enough to make you feel full and energized.

Let's begin with gentle meditation.

Go to a quiet spot and make yourself comfortable. You can lay down or sit, depending on what feels right when you do this. Be prepared to fall asleep. Be at your most comfortable as you close your eyes.

Take a deep breath as you pull your lungs up, and slowly breathe out as you tell yourself to relax completely.

Repeat breathing deeply and by the end of it, tell yourself one more time to relax completely.

Take another deep breath in, fill your lungs with air and hold it for a few seconds before slowly letting it all out. As you do, tell yourself - I'm totally relaxed.

Feel your body as it relaxes completely, following your deep breathing and your words.

Enjoy the feeling of relaxation. Let it flow all the way to your feet.

Now focus on your feet, and feel as they become quite comfortable.

Let the relaxing feeling flow from the feet up to your ankles. Dwell on the feeling.

Continue letting the relaxing feeling flow from your ankles to your leg muscles. Focus on making all the muscles and ligaments in the legs relax completely.

Bring the relaxing sensation up to your knees as you continue breathing deeply. Feel your knees, and your whole body feels utmost relaxation with every exhale.

Let your thighs relax, and gradually bring it up to your hips, then on to your tummy.

As you get a deeper relaxation feeling with each exhale, let it travel to your back. Feel all the muscles become loose and free of tension. Let them sag.

Bring the sensation to your shoulders, over them, and onto your chest.

Now let the relaxing feeling flow into the muscles of your arms, onto your elbows, wrists, and hands, up to each end of your fingertips.

Continue moving the relaxing sensation up to your neck, on your head, and then over it. Let it trickle into your eyebrows, eyes, cheeks, and chin. Unclench your teeth, and allow your jaw to sag.

With each exhale of your breath, feel your entire body relaxing, deeper and deeper.

Count to three, and make your body relax more and more at each count.

Follow the voice. Go deeper into relaxation; the more relaxed you go, the better you feel.

Go even deeper, in a much more relaxed state as you count to five. At each count, feel doubly relaxed from your head to the tip of your toes.

Feel your body, with each organ, each tissue, each fiber, and all your body parts have gone into a deeper state of relaxation.

You are now feeling sleepy. Don't fight it. Relax and let yourself go.

Savor the deeply relaxing feeling as you breathe in and breathe out. Take as much time as you need as you go deeper and deeper.

Breathe in and purposely breathe out. You will now tense your entire body.

Start with your toes - make them tensed. Feel your hands and turn them into fists.

Make each body part tensed as you squeeze tight.

Breathe in and let go of the tension. Allow yourself to feel completely relaxed.

Savor how good relaxation feels.

Now focus on your mind. Free it from any thoughts, and allow it to drift away. Let your mind drift to a far, far away place. Let it go to a place where you feel safe and completely relaxed. Imagine what this place is like, a place where you feel happy and comfortable.

Let your mind drift to a place that feels right at this moment. Enjoy the feeling. Be present at the moment without caring about anything else.

You are lying comfortably as you get yourself in the essence of your being. You are feeling dreamy, warm, and utterly comfortable.

Smell the fresh scent of antiseptics. Smell the fresh linen of a hospital.

Accept that you will undergo a complete change today - that you will be different upon waking up and feel different. You are about to begin a new life.

Feel the hand on your wrist, and visualize the friendly faces of the doctors and nurses at the sides of the trolley where you are lying.

Feel as if the trolley is being moved while you are only vaguely aware of the noises surrounding you. Imagine the ceiling lights as the trolley continue to roll.

Allow yourself to sink deeper as everything becomes more quiet and more calm, as you develop a sense of expectation.

Imagine yourself in a room with a big hospital light above you. But nothing matters. You don't care.

Continue drifting as you go into a deeper sense of relaxation.

Feel your happiness as you realize that today is the day. It is getting done.

In a Nutshell

It's a long chapter tackling the hypnosis techniques you can use to lose weight.

- You have to learn and start performing the techniques, so you will be prepared mentally and emotionally when you start the physical aspects of losing weight.
- Hypnosis aims to reach the unconscious mind to evoke something positive.
- The typical hypnosis techniques used in weight loss are reframing, mind disassociation, changing perspectives, awareness of needs, and gastric band hypnosis.
- Reframing makes it easier for you to stand by your beliefs. This way, you can firmly say no to the temptations of food because you are certain that you are full, you don't eat junk food, and you are never too tired to exercise. Reframing allows you to think whatever you want and become that person.
- Mind disassociation is the technique used by hypnotherapists to change your perspectives about things. It allows you to separate who you are from your thoughts and become an observer to understand things from an outsider's perspective.

- Changing perspectives will give you an alternative reality. Hypnosis aims to open your mind to more possibilities and unchain yourself from old beliefs.
- Awareness of needs talks to your subconscious to prompt it to ask questions instead of questioning things. Not because something has always been like that means that it's right.
- The gastric band hypnosis is specifically designed for weight loss. The concept is similar to gastric bypass surgery, but no surgery will happen. Everything will only be on your mind.

Let's start getting physical in the next chapter. I'll discuss the activities you can do to help you lose weight fast. Let's begin with yoga since it still involves meditation.

CHAPTER EIGHT

Maximizing Your Power and Boosting Your Wellbeing through Yoga

You didn't gain all your weight in one day; you won't lose

it in one day. Be patient with yourself.

- Jenna Wolfe

It's time to be active. But we will take it slow by focusing on yoga exercises. Being active doesn't necessarily mean big movements or too much sweat.

The practice of yoga has gone through a lot of changes and adapted to the needs of its practitioners and those interested in learning more about it. One thing that remains the same is the goal – to unite life's inner and outer qualities.

Yoga is sometimes performed in religious practices, but this is not a religious system. It is a system of exercises and physical poses that will help improve your health and general wellbeing.

It involves varying techniques, poses, and practices to help you become one with the universe. It unifies your mind, body, and spirit until you get to the state of enlightenment.

When done right, yoga can give you the following benefits:

1. Weight loss

It's meditative, but yoga is a form of exercise. It improves your flexibility. You will notice a big difference in how your body can follow even the most difficult yoga poses as you continue practicing. It also makes your bones and muscles stronger. The continued practice also leads to better body posture.

2. Boosts your emotional and spiritual wellbeing

As you burn calories while doing the yoga exercises, it also addresses your emotional and spiritual wellbeing. As you have learned in the previous chapters, the causes of your weight gain may be more complex than you thought. They may be rooted inside you, which yoga can help you understand and address.

3. Good for your health

Since it involves a lot of stretching, yoga protects your spine through well-balanced asana practice. It boosts your blood flow by getting more oxygen into your system. In doing so, it decreases your risk of suffering from heart attack and stroke.

Consistent yoga practice will lower your resting heart rate and boost your endurance.

4. Helps you stay focused

Yoga involves concentration. This is why it is recommended to practice somewhere peaceful and safe. It teaches you how to focus and stay focused during the exercise.

5. Relaxing

It encourages you to relax and let go of the negative vibes.

Yoga is a mind and body practice that allows you to utilize mental and physical disciplines while finding peace and obtaining physical fitness. There are three core components of yoga – poses, breathing, and meditation.

While you can do yoga on your own, finding a trainer who will supervise and guide you initially is better. Joining yoga classes can also expand your world by meeting new people and friends. However, you can opt to do it on your own if that's what you prefer. Make sure you have all the props ready to make the exercises safe. Study the movements before you begin.

MUDRAS AND BASIC POSES

The two of the most useful physical aspect of yoga that can help you lose weight are mudras and asanas. Yoga practice is all about who you are. It helps bring out and understand your core. It guides you to naturally evolve to higher stages of understanding and living life.

Every human being has a physical and non-physical existence that comes in different layers. Yoga aims to activate the principles that will hone each of your layers. The physical practices of yoga are dealt with by learning more about asanas, mudras, and bandhas. They are the three major ways in yoga in which your physical state and spirit are joined.

Asanas are the physical poses, postures, and seats you will learn to improve the spiritual growth of your nervous system, especially the central spinal nerve. On the other hand, mudras are composed of physical and dynamic poses geared towards the parts that channel the flow of the neurobiological energies from your core.

Asanas are known worldwide and integrated with various exercises and physical fitness activities. They help in keeping yoga popular and relevant. Once you have mastered the right poses, it is only natural to learn more about the concept and how you can benefit from it. This leads to finding out more about the other yoga methods, breathing techniques, and practices.

Mudras and bandhas are separate practices with similarities and overlapping techniques. They are done inward, and they train the natural physical processes inside you to help awaken the Kundalini or the point where you will experience spiritual ecstasy.

More about the Mudras in Yoga

A mudra is a gesture typically done using your hands. It directs you to what you must focus on. Mudras come in many kinds and have existed since ancient times. They are also called seals because the movements involve the connection of two parts of your hand. The goal is to create prana or pathways for energy, which you can attain after you have unblocked the chakras.

Mudras have healing effects because of the reflexology points and acupressure found in the hands. Certain mudras do not only heal but are also symbolic. All the aspects of yoga, including mudras, need the practice to benefit from them. However, mudras and other yoga poses and sequences will not work if you don't do them consistently.

The fingers and toes are believed to be charged with divine power in yoga. Each gesture is called a mudra or seal, a hand pantomime done based on the rituals. The mudra carries a visual message similar to a hieroglyph.

After completing a mudra, it symbolically means that you have surrendered yourself. It signifies your commitment. When done during meditation (pranayama), the mudra seals the prana. It directs the prana to your body by preventing it from leaking through your fingers. With the fixed hand pose, you will notice that your brain has become calm, and your fingers are no longer restless.

Mudras can be done in any kind of yoga, and you can do the poses anywhere. They are best performed when doing relaxation and meditation poses.

Here are the common mudras that are typically used in Hatha yoga:

1. Anjali Mudra

This is the most common position, also referred to as the prayer or Namaste position. To do this, firmly press your left palm with your right palm as if you are praying. It's a simple pose, but when done right, it will bring calmness. It is perceived to bring your brain's right and left sides in harmony.

2. Vishnu Mudra

The pose is typically done when performing alternate nostril breathing (Nadi Sodhana). Put your index and middle fingers in the direction of your palm. While the two fingers are bent, keep the rest of the fingers extended.

3. Gyan Mudra

Relax your fingers. Bring your thumb and forefinger closer and press them firmly while the remaining fingers are left lying straight. If you are doing this mudra in a cross-legged pose, allow the backs of your hands to lie on your thighs comfortably. This is called knowledge mudra (Jnana mudra) and symbolizes connection and oneness.

4. Lotus Mudra

Start with both of your palms touching, like in Anjali mudra. Do not allow your thumbs, pinkies, and the bases of your palms to disconnect as you separate the middle parts of your palms and spread the rest of the fingers. Once done, the pose looks similar to the shape of a lotus flower. Like a flower, this mudra symbolizes openness and blossoming.

5. Garuda Mudra

The pose has a balancing and invigorating effect, same as its origin, the eagle pose or Garudasana. The pose will remind you of a bird. Cross your wrists with your palms in the direction of your chest. Hook the thumbs of your two hands together.

6. Dhyana Mudra

It's a classic Buddhist meditation pose. While sitting down, lay your left hand on your lap with the palm facing up. Put your right hand on top of the left. Let your thumbs get in contact above your palms as you do this.

7. Kundalini Mudra

The pose is connected with one's sexuality and unity. Form a fist with your left hand while keeping the index finger extended. Grip that index finger with your right hand as you make a fist with this hand. Keep the thumb of your right hand lying on top of the index finger of your left hand.

Yoga Poses and Mudras for Beginners

Let's do the mudras and the basic yoga poses you can perform together. You can begin with the following basic poses. Be mindful of your hand gestures or mudras as you do the poses:

1. Toe stand (Pandangustasana)

If you have knee pain, do a couple of minutes of hip stretching before you begin. This pose helps open the hips and make the core of the feet stronger. Stand in a half lotus tree pose. Stand on your right leg and move the top of your left foot towards your right hip. Breathe deeply to keep your balance.

Slowly bend your right knee while keeping your left foot on the left thigh. Lift your right heel until you are up on the ball of your right foot. As you go on a squat, do your best so that the right heel will be in the center of your body. Aiming the right heel under the right buttock is a common mistake.

Extend your fingertips to the floor ahead of you to attain more balance. Make your belly firm as you try to lift one hand or both, if you can, off the floor. Keep your balance on the ball of your right foot. Once you have achieved the perfect balance, move your hands and perform Anjali mudra. Hold the pose as you inhale and exhale deeply for five counts.

Start getting out of the pose by returning to the half lotus tree pose. You will do the same to the other side, but shake both legs before you continue. If your hips find it hard to follow the sequence, focus on attaining your balance in a squat with your heels lifted and your knees together. You will eventually get this right and easy.

2. Revolved lunge

This is a detoxifying pose that requires flexibility, balance, and strength. It is detoxifying because it involves doing a twist that will wring your internal organs and give your chest enough room to breathe by the end of the pose.

Start with a regular lunge pose with your hands down. Twist to the right by stepping your left foot backward. You will get to a high lunge pose with your knee directly facing your ankle and all your toes facing forward. Make your weight stable to attain balance by reaching through the back heel. Bring your hands to Anjali mudra in front of your chest and perform a twist to the right.

Place your elbow and press it outside of the knee. Put your hands together and place them in the middle part of your chest. It's normal if you can't put your elbow down to your knee in the beginning. Constant practice will help you get used to it. If you still can't perform the pose properly, you can retain one hand in the prayer position while the other arm is extended.

If you can't keep your balance, keep the back of your knee down with your toes tucked underneath. As a beginner, keeping your lower back safe is more important than performing the movements perfectly. You can choose to perform the twist in a low lunge or twisting your rib cage. Make sure that the belly button is up as you twist. Keep your chin tucked as you reach the crown of your head.

Go back to the lunge position with your hands down to come out of the pose. Step forward and roll up as gently as you can.

3. Deep side lunge (Skandasana)

Begin with a wide-legged forward bend (Prasarita Padottanasana). Gently bend your knee until you are on a half squat. Ensure your right leg remains straight as you extend your foot and let your toes leave the floor. Rest your weight on your right heel. You can keep your hands on the floor, especially if you are finding it hard to keep your balance.

As you become more used to the practice, you can bend your elbows as you bring your hands together to an Anjali mudra pose, with your left elbow kept at the inner part of the left knee. Drop your hands to the floor for support to come off the pose. Gradually shift and perform the actions to the other side.

Beginners are not expected to get into a full squat. It takes practice and getting used to. While you are still trying to perfect the pose, you can stay up on the ball of the left foot.

After familiarizing yourself with the basic and easier poses, you can explore other yoga practices. As you continue practicing yoga and as the poses become more challenging, you will start reaping the benefits of the practice. It brings you calm while also helping you with your goal of losing weight quickly and efficiently.

Practicing the More Challenging Yoga Mudras

The yoga mudras have a direct relationship with the five elements of the human body. This concept is further explained in Ayurveda. According to Ayurveda, there is an imbalance in the body when you suffer from a disease. The imbalance can either be due to the lack or excess of the five elements.

You can find the characteristics of these five elements in your fingers, making your fingers important electrical circuits. You will use the mudras to adjust the flow of energy that significantly affects the balance of water, earth, air, fire, and ether to imbibe healing.

Here are the other mudras you can start practicing on. Before you begin, make sure that you are in a comfortable position. You can either sit on a chair or get into certain yoga poses, such as cross-legged or lotus.

1. Chin mudra

Hold the thumb and your forefinger lightly while the rest of the fingers remain extended and straight. Place your hands on top of your thighs, with the palms facing up, and wait until you have established your breathing. Relax your fingers and focus on your breathing. Observe how the process and flow of your breathing affect you.

2. Chinmaya mudra

Form a ring with your thumb and forefinger, and let the three remaining fingers curl in your palm. Place your hands on your thighs, with palms facing up. Take deep ujjayi breaths, but make sure you remain comfortable throughout the process. You will need to focus on your breathing and its effects.

3. Adi mudra

Place your thumb at the base of your small finger while the rest of the fingers are curled over the thumb in a light fist. Put your hands on your thighs, with palms facing up, breathe deeply, and observe the effects.

4. Brahma mudra

Place both hands in the position that you have done in Adi Mudra. Put the knuckles of your hands together and place them in the navel area as you keep on breathing and observing its flow. Take at least 12 breaths to observe the effects clearly. Focus and be mindful of where your breath is flowing and how it affects your mind and body.

The Eight Basic Hand Gestures Used in Yoga and Meditation

There are two basic kinds of mudras in yoga. One involves touching the tips of different fingers with the thumb. The second one is pressing the first phalangeal joint with the thumb. Their effects will depend on which fingers are touching or being pressed. This is because the body is composed of special points targeted by acupressure and acupuncture to heal.

The first two mudras below affect the air, the first of the five elements of your body. It is responsible for your mental health, creativity, and intellect and is associated with Anahata or the fourth chakra.

1. Gyan mudra (Vaayu Vardhak)

Vaayu means air, and Cardhak means to enhance. This mudra affects one's wisdom.

Touch the tips of your index finger with the thumb. In professional yoga, practitioners do this to meditate and disassociate themselves from the material world. It helps in increasing the element of air in the body. It prompts your creative thinking, enthusiasm, and eagerness.

It can help improve your memory and boost the cognitive process of thinking when done consistently. It can also alleviate depression, drowsiness, and mental retardation. You can practice this mudra anytime and anywhere you are.

2. Vaayu mudra (Vaayu Shaamak)

Vaayu means air, and Shaamak means to suppress. This mudra soothes your emotions and makes you feel calm. Put the tip of your index finger at the base of your thumb; thumb upon this finger and carefully press it.

This mudra decreases the air element in your body, which in effect, soothes your spirit and calms your mind. It works by soothing your nervous system and any kind of hormonal imbalance. This is a recommended activity for hyperactive and aggressive people and those who have difficulty keeping their focus.

The next mudras affect the second element of the human body, the ether or space, which is subtle and mostly inactive. It is responsible for your collective consciousness and allows you to resonate with the cosmos. It is mainly associated with Visudda or the fifth chakra.

3. Aakash mudra

The term means Aakash or space and Vardhak or to enhance. It gives you the feeling of lightness. Gently touch the tips of the middle finger with the thumb. The gesture boosts the space element in your body. It eases away your negative thoughts and worries. It also helps you deal with anger, sadness, and fear. It has a detoxifying effect and is ideal for people who frequently suffer from congestion problems in the tummy, ear, sinus, and chest.

For best results, perform this mudra early in the morning or in the afternoon. Make sure you don't do it longer than 30 minutes each day if you have a weak body.

4. Shunya mudra (Aakash Shaamak)

Aakash means space, and Shaamak means to suppress. This mudra has a healing effect on pains. Touch the tip of your middle finger at the base of your thumb and thumb upon this finger by carefully pressing it.

It decreases the space element in your body and helps relieve ear-related pains, such as minor aches, tinnitus, impaired hearing, travel sickness, and nausea. It also prevents numbness in your chest and head. This is recommended for people who have a pronounced Vata constitution. You can do this anytime, but if you are performing this mudra to get rid of ear aches, numbness and vertigo, stop it when you feel that the pain has subsided.

The next mudras are targeted at the Earth element of the human body, which is responsible for the physical construction, such as the bones and tissues. This element also governs your nose. The chakra that is associated with the earth element is the first kind, which is Muladhara.

They also address the fire element that controls the body's glands, metabolism, growth, and temperature. The fire element is associated with the third chakra, the Manipura.

5. Prithvi mudra (Prithvi Vardhak)

Prithvi means earth, and Vardhak means to enhance. It is also called Agni Shaamak Mudra. Agni means fire, and Shaamak means to suppress. This mudra affects one's strength. Touch the tips of your ring finger to your thumb.

The action decreases the fire element in your body while boosting the earth element. It allows you to heal, build muscles, and encourage new tissue growth. It helps boost your energy and is effective for those suffering from dry skin and brittle nails, hair, and bones. It promotes endurance and vitality. This also works by regulating your body temperature and metabolic process.

6. Surya mudra (Prithvi Shaamak)

Prithvi means earth, and Shaamak means to suppress. It is also called Agni Vardhak Mudra. Agni means fire, and Vardhak means to enhance. Place the tip of the ring finger at the base of the thumb. You will thumb upon that finger by gently pressing it.

It works by decreasing the earth element while increasing the fire element in your system. This is recommended when you are shivering due to low temperature and colds. It can help you lose weight as it aids digestion. It also enables you to feel better if you have constipation, suffer from a lack of appetite and suppressed thyroid activity. This can be done any time during the day, but do not exceed 30 minutes for each session because it can cause your body to overheat.

Water is the body's fifth and final element, making up more than 70 percent of the human body. It influences your skin, tongue, taste, tissues, and joints. It corresponds to the second chakra, the energy chakra called Swadhisthana.

7. Varun mudra (Jal Vardhak)

Jal means war, and Vardhak means to enhance. Gently touch the tips of the little finger with your thumb.

This mudra works by increasing the water element in your body. It has a moisturizing effect and is recommended for those suffering from general dehydration, cramps, and hormonal deficiency. It relieves joint pains, arthritis and improves the condition of those who have lost the sensation of taste and experience limited body secretions.

This works wonders for people with dry hair, eyes, and skin and those suffering from digestive health problems and eczema. This is safe for everybody except for people with water retention problems.

8. Jal Shaamak mudra

Jal means water, and Shaamak means to suppress. This action is intended for stability. Put the tip of your little finger to the base of the thumb and thumb upon that finger by gently pressing it.

It works by decreasing the water element in the body. This is recommended for people with problems with water retention or edema, hyperacidity, too much glandular secretion, watery eyes, sweaty palms, runny nose, and salivation.

THE ASANAS

The asanas have been adapted to the physical fitness industry. Asanas or physical postures are essential in executing the other styles of yoga. They are defined by types, benefits, anatomy, and many more.

Many kinds of asanas depend on your initial pose upon doing the exercise and what you aim to achieve. These poses include standing, arm balance, balancing, binding, chest opening, core yoga poses, forward bend, hip opening, inversion, pranayama, restorative, seated, strengthening, twist, backbends, and bandha.

Let's begin your introduction to yoga by doing standing yoga poses.

1. Big Toe Pose (Padangusthasana)

Stand straight with the inner part of your feet parallel and almost six inches apart from each other. Lift your kneecaps by contracting the front muscles of your thigh. Breathe out while ensuring that your legs remain straight and perform a forward bend from the hip joints to your torso and head.

Slide the index and middle fingers of your two hands in the center of the big toes and the second toes. Curl your fingers under and get a firm grip with your big toes. Wrap the thumbs around the other two fingers to make the grip more secure. You will then press the toes against the fingers. If you find it hard to reach your toes without exerting too much effort on your back, you can pass straps beneath the balls of your feet and hold onto the straps instead.

As you inhale, you will lift your torso as if you are going to stand up by extending your elbows. Stretch the front part of your torso, exhale and lift your sitting bones. Release your hamstrings and hollow the part below your navel to lift it slightly towards the back part of your pelvis.

While keeping your forehead relaxed, lift your sternum as high as possible. Ensure you don't overdo the action of compressing the back of your neck.

Inhale as you lift your torso strong while you continue to contract your front thighs. On the next exhalations, lift your sitting bones with force while you allow your hamstrings to relax. Make sure that you make the hollow in your lower back deeper.

Exhale and bend your elbows to the sides. Pull up on your toes and stretch the front and sides of your torso. Gently lower the torso by doing a forward bend.

Hold the position for one minute. Lose the grip on your toes, put your hands to your hips and stretch your front torso. Inhale and swing your torso and head as if you are dealing with a single unit as you go back to an upright pose.

2. Mountain Pose (Tadasana)

Stand straight with the bases of your big toes touching and the second toes parallel. Lift and spread your toes, move the balls of your feet, and slowly put them back to the floor. Begin rocking your weight by moving your feet to the front and back and then from side to side. Gradually reduce the frequency of the swaying of your body until you are standing still and your feet are carrying your weight in a balanced manner.

Lift your kneecaps while ensuring that your thigh muscles remain firm and your lower belly is relaxed. Lift the inner parts of your ankles. Envision that there is a line of energy from your inner thighs to the groins, going through the core of your torso, neck, and crown of your head. Move the upper parts of your thighs inward. Extend your tailbone to the floor and lift your pubis toward the navel.

Keep the shoulder blades in the back, begin to spread them across, and gently release them down your back. Lift the top part of the sternum toward the ceiling while ensuring that your ribs are not pushed forward. Spread your collarbones while you let your arms hang at each side of your torso.

Make sure that the crown of your head is balanced. The underside of your chin has to be parallel to the floor, your tongue is wide and flat to the mouth, and the throat and your gaze remain soft. This is the usual starting position of the standing poses.

3. Dolphin Pose

The position opens your shoulders and works on your core, arms, and legs. Come down on the floor on your hands and knees, with your knees below the hips, your forearms on the floor, and your shoulders above your wrists. Press your palms together in a firm manner.

Curl your toes, exhale and begin lifting your knees in a slightly bent manner and the heels lifted away from the floor. Extend your tailbone in the opposite direction of the back of your pelvis, and press it slightly to your pubis. As you feel the resistance at this point, begin lifting the sitting bones upward. Draw your inner legs up to your groins.

Keep your forearms pressed to the floor while your shoulder blades are firm against the back. Extend the blades and draw them near your tailbone. Keep your head between the upper arms; do not allow it to hang or get pressed against the floor. It is okay to straighten your knees if the position is becoming uncomfortable. Keep extending your tailbone away from the pelvis. Lift the upper part of the sternum away from the floor. Stay in this position for up to a minute. Release your knees as you exhale.

4. Chair Pose (Utkatasana)

The position utilizes the muscles in your legs and arms, which benefits your heart and diaphragm.

Begin by standing in Tadasana. Breathe in as you move your arms upwards until they are perpendicular to the floor. Keep your arms parallel with the palms facing inward. Slowly bend your knees as you exhale. Try to position your thighs as nearly parallel to the floor as your body will allow you to. This will push your torso slightly forward until it forms a right angle with the top parts of the thighs. Make sure that the inner thighs remain parallel to one another as you press the heads of the bones of your thighs in the direction of your heels.

Relax your shoulder blades and allow them to get firm against your back. Move your tailbone towards the floor and to your pubis while keeping the lower part of the back long. Hold the position for up to a minute. Inhale as you begin straightening your knees and lifting through your arms. Release your arms and put them on each side as you exhale and return to Tadasana.

5. Downward-Facing Dog (Adho Mukha Svanasana)

This is among the most popular yoga poses because it exercises the whole body and gives you a rejuvenating stretch. Begin with your hands and knees to the floor. Spread your palms, turn your toes, and keep your knees below your hips.

Gently lift your knees as you exhale. At first, keep the knees a little bent and the heels lifted. Extend your tailbone from behind your pelvis and press it toward the pubis. As you feel the resistance, lift the sitting bones and draw your inner legs towards the groins.

Push the top parts of your thighs as you exhale and extend your heels to the floor. Straighten the knees without locking them. Make the muscles of the thighs firm as you roll the upper parts slightly inward. Make the front of the pelvis narrow.

Keep the bases of the index fingers pressed to the floor while the outer arms are firm. Lift the inner arms towards your upper shoulders while ensuring that the shoulder blades remain firm behind the back. Extend your shoulder blades and draw them into the tailbone while your head remains between your upper arms.

6. Extended Hand-To-Big-Toe Pose (Utthita Hasta Padangustasana)

Start in a Tadasana pose, and bring your left knee near your tummy. Extend your left arm and try to reach the inner part of your thigh. Cross your left arm over your front ankle and keep it outside the left. You can opt to loop a strap on your left sole and hold onto it if you feel that your hamstrings are tight.

Make the front part of your thigh muscles firm as you press the outer thigh inward. As you inhale, stretch your left leg in front while keeping your knee as straight as possible. Once you are steady, begin swinging the left leg to the side. As you perform the movements, make steady breathing because it requires concentration while helping you to maintain your balance.

Hold the pose for 30 seconds, and then swing the leg back to the middle as you inhale. When you exhale, begin lowering your foot to the floor. Repeat the sequences to the other side.

7. Eagle Pose (Garudasana)

This pose effectively gives you endurance, concentration, flexibility, and strength. You will begin with the Tadasana pose. Slightly curve your knees and move your left foot toward the ceiling. Keep the right foot balanced as the left thigh crosses over the other. Position the left toes parallel to the floor while you press the foot and hook the upper part of the foot at the back of the lower right calf. Maintain your balance using your right foot.

Extend your arms, spreading the scapulas across the back part of the torso. Put the right arm at the top of the left, in front of your torso, and begin bending your elbows. Put the right elbow into the corner of the left elbow and extend the forearms until they are positioned vertically to the mat. Make sure that the back parts of your hands are facing one another.

Move the palms so that they are already facing each other. Allow the thumb of the right hand to move beyond the little finger of your left hand. With as much force as possible, press your palms together, lift your elbows, and spread your fingers upwards. Keep the position for up to 30 seconds. You will then unwind your arms and legs and return to the Tadasana pose. Repeat the sequence using the other sides of your legs and arms.

8. Extended Side Angle Pose (Utthita Parsvakonasana)

Begin in a Tadasana pose. As you exhale, step your feet up to four feet apart. Extend the arms parallel to the floor as you move each of them towards your sides with your palms facing down and your shoulder blades wide.

Slightly move your left foot to the right and the right foot to the right at a 90-degree angle. Keep the right and left heels aligned. While keeping the thighs firm, turn the right thigh outward until the middle of the kneecap is aligned with the middle of the right ankle. Slightly roll your left hip forward and then to the right as you rotate the upper part of the torso to the left.

Lift the inner part of the left groin deep into your pelvis to anchor the left heel to the floor. As you exhale, start bending the right knee over the right ankle. This will make your shin perpendicular to the floor.

Make your shoulder blades firm against the back of your ribs. Stretch your left arm upwards, turn the left palm in the direction of your head and inhale as you reach the arm towards the back of your left ear with your palm facing the floor. Extend your left heel as you lengthen the left side of your body. Make your head turn in the direction of your left arm, and release the right shoulder away from the ear. Create equal length along both sides of your torso.

When you exhale, put the right side of your torso down to the top of your right thigh. Press your palm on the floor near the outer part of your right foot. Keep pushing your right knee against the inner part of the arm while you create tension by putting your tailbone to the back of your pelvis in the direction of the pubis. At this point, the inner part of your right thigh must be parallel to the long edge of your mat.

Hold the pose up to a minute. Inhale as you begin to come up. Push your heels to the floor with force and extend the left arm forcefully upwards. Reverse the position of your feet and repeat the sequence. Return to the Tadasana pose when you are done.

9. Standing Half Forward Bend (Ardha Uttanasana)

Begin with a standing forward bend or Uttanasana. Press your fingertips to the floor beside your feet, or you can press your palms if you can. As you inhale, stretch your elbows and move your torso away from your thighs. Try your best to widen the length between the navel and pubic bone.

Using the strength coming from your fingertips or palms, begin lifting the top part of your sternum and moving it forward. If you find it more comfortable, you can slightly bend your knees, which will cause your back to arch.

Look in front of you without compressing the back of your neck. Hold the pose for several breaths, exhale and release your torso to full Uttanasana.

10.   Extended   Triangle   Pose   (Utthita Trikonasana)

Begin in the Tadasana pose. Exhale and step until your feet are up to four feet apart. Extend your arms, keeping them parallel to the floor, and actively reach the sides with your palms down and the shoulder blades wide. Slightly turn the left foot to the right direction and the right foot out to the right at a 90-degree angle. Keep both heels aligned. Make the thighs firm as you turn the right thigh outward until the middle of the right kneecap is parallel to the middle of your right ankle.

Exhale and stretch your torso to the right as you bend from the hip joint. Strengthen the left leg as you perform the movement and press the outer part of the leg steadily to the floor. Perform a torso rotation to the left while the two sides remain equally long. Allow your hip to come forward slightly as you extend the tailbone to the back heel.

Let your right hand rest on your shin or the floor outside of the right foot. Extend your left arm upward while keeping it in line with the top parts of the shoulders. Your head should be in a neutral position as you turn it to the left and allow your gaze to focus on your left thumb. Keep the pose up to a minute. Come up as you inhale while pressing the back heel firmly to the floor and reaching the top part of your arm in the direction of the ceiling. Perform the same sequence after you have reversed the feet.

In a Nutshell

After understanding your core and what's happening inside you, it's time to be active. This chapter introduces you to yoga.

- Yoga is a system of exercises and physical poses that promotes well-being.
- Yoga has many benefits, one of which is weight loss. It's a form of meditation and exercise.
- The most beneficial physical aspects of yoga to help you lose weight are mudras and asanas.
- Mudras are gestures done using the hands. They create prana or pathways for energy that you can benefit from after you have unlocked the chakras.

- Mudras are healing and symbolic. They are better done together with yoga poses.
- The asanas are the physical poses defined by types, benefits, anatomy, and more.
- There are many asana poses, but this chapter introduced you to ten basic poses you can follow to begin learning about yoga.

Let us learn more about the benefits of being active and what you will do when you feel lethargic or stuck. Head on to the next chapter.

CHAPTER NINE
The Extent of Being Active to Weight Loss

Remember, you have been criticizing yourself for years and it hasn't worked. Try approving of yourself and see what happens.

- Louise Hay

Losing weight is a process. It's a lifetime commitment to fitness and health. Your work doesn't stop once you have obtained your ideal weight. You have to make your newfound love for wellness part of your lifestyle.

Yoga is a good practice that targets the body, mind, and soul. However, you have more options regarding the physical activities you can try to lose weight rapidly and make it easier to stay that way.

You have already dealt with your relationship with food. You have learned to reprogram the signals inside to eliminate emotional, habitual, and compulsive eating. The more energy your release, the faster you will lose weight. It's easier to burn extra energy when doing physical activities. For example, eating a full meal and brisk walking for 30 minutes is better than not doing any physical activity but eating only half of your meal. The latter situation will make you hungry.

Aside from helping you lose weight, being active offers many health benefits. It speeds up your metabolism, which leads to rapid weight loss.

When you are overweight, you are at great risk of certain cancers, diabetes, stroke, heart disease, and high blood pressure. It also makes you prone to joint and bone pains. If inactive for too long, you may become susceptible to osteoporosis. You can counter all these by adopting a more active lifestyle.

Being active will also reduce your stress and bring about positivity. It will help you better deal with sadness or depression without suffering from the side effects of treatments and medications.

More physical activities will result in the body's production of endorphins in the brain. The hormones will make you feel happier and less anxious. Being constantly active will make you feel and look good. It will also help you age well and suffer fewer pains when you age.

How active should you be?

It depends. You should consult your doctor before trying physical exercises or even yoga if you are suffering from certain illnesses. If you are free to become as active as possible, do it and start now. It's easy, but you need to start soon, so you will get used to the activities faster.

An exercise is a form of aerobic activity that makes you warm and breathe harder. It doesn't have to be an actual exercise as long as the activity makes you sweat and breathe deeply.

The aerobic activity allows the body to use more energy and requires your muscles and heart to work harder. It boosts your energy and metabolism.

It helps you lose weight.

GETTING ACTIVE AND FIT - A PERFECT COMBINATION

You can do many activities to become active. You can walk the dog, carry shopping bags, climb the stairs, water the plants, or clean the house. The easiest way to become active is by walking. You can do it anywhere, even inside your house. You can make walking part of your routine, especially when you're off somewhere near and the weather is nice.

You can make this phase of being active more fun as well. You can try doing something rewarding or activities you haven't tried before. You can get a gym membership form or enroll in a yoga class to get fit and meet new people. You can also participate in events, like a marathon or charity walks.

UNDERSTANDING LETHARGY

Lethargy is the general feeling of not wanting to do anything or feeling listless. If you have nurtured this feeling for long without intending to, it may be hard to get free from it. But it has to be done. If not, you will find adapting to a more active lifestyle hard.

You are your worst enemy. Many opportunities may surround you, but without self-discipline and willpower, you are bound to make the wrong choices and fail. This happens when you are stuck to the feeling of being lethargic. It makes your life feel stagnant. But the problem is not with the world. It's you.

Here are the signs that you have fallen into the trap of lethargy:

1. Lack of self-discipline

Self-discipline is like fuel that prompts you to take action to get something done with the right intentions. When you lack discipline, it shows. You tend to do certain things without thinking about how others would feel. And many times, you don't do anything at all.

For example, you did not show up at an invitation of a friend to go biking together even after you have committed. You did not think about what the other person would feel or who would accompany her in biking. By not showing up, your friend would feel disrespected because you did not value your commitment and their time.

You tend to neglect your responsibilities and obligations when you lack self-discipline. You must reassess yourself and find out where the problem lies before this attitude worsens.

2. Attitude and commitment

You have to give importance and give the same amount of respect to every individual, including yourself. Whenever you make a decision, you must think about how it will affect yourself and those around you. You have to see life as something sacred. Every day allows you to prove yourself and attain your goals. You have to do so in ways that you remain considerate and respectful to other people who might be affected by whatever it is you will do.

It is easier to cultivate self-discipline when you appreciate and value life. You will not find it hard to show others love and respect when you love and respect yourself. It prompts you to commit and stay true to it. When you are committed to something, you feel enthusiastic about honoring your commitments.

3. Weaknesses in your character

Life always gives you choices. You can choose to pursue the right thing because you feel good about it or do nothing because you are scared that you cannot keep up with it. When you lack character, you are driven by the wrong motivations, such as power or greed, rather than selflessness and love. You have to learn to love yourself and respect other people.

4. Lack of self-awareness

Most of the time, you are unaware that your negative thoughts are already causing you to self-destruct. The more time you spend thinking about them, the less productive you become. You have to be aware that the negative mind power is already ruining your potential to grow and succeed. You have to stop it by becoming aware that the problem exists.

Thinking negatively may have become a habit that you allowed yourself to succumb to. Whenever you are making a decision, listen to yourself first. You must always be aware of the voice that feeds your mind with negative thoughts. You have to find a way to turn all the negative points into something positive and productive.

5. Lack of desire, passion, and love

Your desire and love to get something done drives you to do it. Without this passion, you will lack the discipline to take action whenever possible. When you lack self-discipline, your actions are provoked by self-interest, power, self-indulgence, and sometimes, anger. This makes you do things without thinking about the repercussions or how they will affect those around you. When you have self-discipline, you do things because there is a willingness to do good and become better.

It becomes your expression of unconditional love for yourself, your goals, and your ambitions.

6. Lack of ambition

The kind of ambition that you have says a lot about your character. In honing your self-discipline, you must also shape the types of ambition born out of respect, grace, and honesty.

7. Wrong Priorities

Whenever you work towards a goal, think about how this will affect your life in general and other people's lives. If you only work for your own good, you might reap success but not genuine happiness. You have to find purpose and the meaning of why you are doing these things.

8. Laziness

It is okay to feel tired every once in a while, but it is different when you are psyching yourself that you are tired due to a lack of self-motivation. If you strongly believe there is a good reason why you need to accomplish your goal, nothing will block your way in doing everything to get to the finish line. When motivated by this belief, you will always feel energetic and have a strong urge to see how things will turn out. You have to get past your laziness by understanding the factors that stop you from carrying out your responsibilities.

9. Lack of self-respect

You don't value yourself or give yourself enough importance to achieve and excel. It all boils down to self-discipline. It drives you to become excellent, keep on getting better, achieve your goals, and set new ones. When you regard yourself highly, and with respect, you don't settle for what is easy. You are always challenging yourself to maximize all the possibilities, live your life to the fullest and achieve your goals without stepping on other people's toes.

It is easier to become productive when you respect yourself. This will also make it easier for you to reach out to others and extend help.

Get Past the Lethargy and Start Controlling Your Life

Just do it. If you want to change for the better, you will no longer wait for another minute to begin with the things you need to do. Think about the lost chances and the severed ties due to your lack of self-discipline.

Set a goal - change your attitude and become more disciplined. Promise yourself that you will stick to the goal and will get things done no matter how hard it may be.

Here are some of the steps that will help you develop your willpower and self-discipline:

1. Practice mindfulness meditation

A few minutes each day of this meditation will help boost your willpower. It is not geared to changing who you are; instead, the meditation helps you become aware of the present and what brought you here.

When you are mindful, you don't contemplate how you wish things are different. Instead, you become aware of what needs to be done, pushing yourself to do it. The more mindful you are, the more compassionate you become towards yourself and the people around you.

Make sure to work on these three aspects when you practice mindfulness meditation – your body, breathing, and mind.

Mind

When new to this practice, you notice that random thoughts keep popping up. You suddenly remember different recollections about your life. This is normal. But when you feel like the thoughts are becoming too empowering, bring your mind to the present. Try hard to focus on your breathing.

The whole practice can be done for 10 to 30 minutes each day. It doesn't prevent you from thinking. The goal is not to clear your mind from any thoughts. It helps you to focus and be mindful of what is happening at the moment.

Body

Go somewhere comfortable and quiet. You can sit on a chair or a cushion on the floor. Keep your posture upright but not stiff. Imagine that your spine is a tree, and then lean against that tree. Cross your legs and place your hands on your thighs. Allow your gaze to linger anywhere in front up to six feet away. Stay put for several minutes. Whenever your mind wanders, gently bring it back to the present.

Breathing

Try to feel your breath as you inhale and exhale. There is no right or wrong way to do this. You are only trying to channel your attention to how you breathe. Appreciate it and observe how you breathe in and breathe out. Spend several minutes on this part of the meditation.

2. Exercise

Keeping yourself physically fit by being active helps improve your mood and mental performance. It also reduces the percentage of your body fat, stress levels, and sleep quality. As you gain more benefits from the activity, you will notice a great improvement in your willpower.

You can begin by doing physical exercises for at least five minutes daily. Start easy by walking around the house, jogging in the backyard, or doing simple stretches at the start of your day. As your body gets used to the habit, you can challenge yourself to perform more physically-draining activities and do the exercises at least 30 minutes thrice a week.

Some people argue that exercising is not for them. There is no such thing as not being made for exercising. You may not have yet found the right exercises you both enjoy and benefit from. Keep trying various physical activities until you find the ones you can stick with as part of your routine.

You can also do it with others to make the experience more enjoyable. You can go to the gym and enroll in aerobics or dance classes. You can also ask a friend to be your exercise partner.

3. Redefine your goals

Why did you lose track of your goals? From now on, you have to live life with a greater purpose. You must know where your life is leading. Set the goals you know you can do. You can always set higher goals but start with the smaller ones. Once you begin reaping the fruits of your labor, it will push you to become better and to obtain more.

4. Stop making excuses

You always have to feel accountable for your every action. You have to start living your life with higher standards. Your motto in life from now on must be no more excuses. This will prevent you from making excuses whenever you feel like you cannot keep up with your commitment.

5. Stay away from temptations

Get rid of any temptations that might distract you from achieving your goals. You know your weaknesses, so make sure that you avoid them whenever you are determined to finish something. Do not give yourself any reasons to come up with any more excuses. Identify the everyday distractions and work your way to build a structure to block these off.

6. Focus

Focus on the more essential things. When you make a decision, make sure that this is not only for your own good but will benefit other people or the other aspects of your life. Do not spend a lot of time thinking about something trivial.

7. Honor your commitments

Give your 100 percent commitment all the time. Avoid listening to the inner voice that tells you to slow down or take a break when you have a responsibility to carry on. It takes efficient willpower to win over this thought and say that you can and will do it.

8. Be positive

Make it a habit to live your life with a positive outlook. Always begin your day thinking good things will happen and end it by looking forward to another great day. Make this part of your lifestyle.

From here on, you must push yourself, especially when you feel like backing out. Focus on the present. Do what needs to be done and move forward.

A Meditation to Break Free from Lethargy

Here's a meditation technique you can use to realize you're under the power of lethargy and do something to break free from it:

Go somewhere quiet and be comfortable. Remember the last time you wanted to exercise but felt too disinterested to start anything. Imagine what you did and how you looked at that point. Imagine how you felt when you couldn't push yourself to exercise. Hold on to that thought.

Think of someone you look up to when it comes to fitness. Imagine that person shaking you up. Think about how you would feel if only you were that person. If only you could be more determined and motivated, you could follow that person's lead. Now imagine yourself having the determination and motivation to be that person.

Close your eyes. Visualize that in front of you is a picture of your old lethargic self. Imagine the picture getting brighter and bigger. Now visualize a small picture beside the image. It's the new you - the motivated and determined person. But the picture is dark and small. Swap the images real quick. Make the positive picture brighter and bigger, and the old picture darker and smaller. Imagine the photos fading away, and open your eyes.

You will repeat the visualization of the picture swapping. Open your eyes every time they have faded away. Make sure that you swap fast. Repeat until you have gotten to the point that you can no longer remember what the old picture looks like.

When you have gotten to the point, you will feel renewed and have the determination to start getting active.

Close your eyes. Visualize a time when you will go out to exercise. How do you look and feel? If your look determined and motivated, savor that and allow that image you see to become more appealing. Keep it going as you form a fist in your left hand and squeeze it. Relax your hand and open your eyes.

If you did not see the motivated image of yourself when you visualize, you have to repeat the step of picture swapping and try again.

Squeezing your fist is like a reminder for yourself to keep the motivation and maximize the power you've got from doing the meditation.

HOW TO BECOME MORE CONFIDENT ABOUT YOURSELF?

It is easier to keep up with your plans, show up, and make people believe that you can do things when you exude the aura that you can do it. Aside from loving yourself, you also have to develop self-confidence. It may come easily once you have started losing weight. But you don't have to wait until you get to that goal.

Here are some tips on how you can boost your self-belief and confidence:

1. Turn the negative into positive

Always replace negative thoughts with positive ones. It is only natural for your mind to wander and wonder about what other people are saying behind your back. Do not spend too much time thinking and sulking about these petty things. There are more important things that you need to focus on. Always step forward with a positive vibe.

2. Look the part

Project the image that you want other people to see in you. You have to picture what you want your image to be, then work your way to make that image come to life. Take a shower, shave or sport a nice haircut. Fill your closet with good clothes. Never go out without looking presentable. You are not drastically changing who you are. You are only claiming the kind of life you deserve and that you have chosen to avoid for a long time.

3. Know who you are

You have to understand your strengths and weaknesses and learn how to balance the two. Focus on your strengths, especially when you feel you are being tested. Think about your limitations. Challenge yourself and prove that you can get past them.

4. Empower yourself

Never stop learning to add new skills and widen your knowledge. Keep on reading and always be informed about the news and trends around you. This will make it easier for you to talk to different people. This will also make you more confident when you are presenting something to a group of people or your bosses.

5. Exude confidence

Whenever you approach people, do it in a way that they will feel your aura. Put your positive energy into everything that you do. This will make it easier for you to accomplish things you thought you could not do. Part of becoming more positive is by spreading good vibes. You have to start being kind to yourself and other people.

6. Smile

Do not let it show whenever you feel afraid, nervous, or beaten. Smile, and you will feel better. By keeping a genuine smile plastered on your lips, other people will be drawn to you, and you will be kinder to them as well.

7. Speak slowly and eloquently

When you speak, make sure that people will listen because they find you interesting and understand what you are saying. People with low self-esteem will try to speak quickly and softly. They think that no one would care about what they have to say or that they are not worth listening to. You have to speak in a manner that gives other people the impression that it is worth listening to every word you say.

8. Instead of complaining, look for solutions

You are only making your problems worse when you constantly complain. You have to focus on how to get rid of the problems and do them.

9. Volunteer

Volunteer whenever you have time. It will make you feel better about yourself when you see how you make other people happy by sharing your time and effort. This will also make your life more valuable. You are beginning to live not only for your own good but also for the sake of those who need your help.

10. Develop a good posture

Your confidence shows in how you carry yourself. You must stand tall and always maintain a good posture.

HOW TO MAKE IT EASIER TO BECOME MORE ACTIVE?

You can be more active no mate your age or work. There is no such thing as too busy (or too lazy). You can find time as long as you want what you will do. So in becoming more active, make the activities more convenient, enjoyable, and engaging.

The US Department of Health and the UK Chief Medical Officer suggest adults exercise 150 minutes each week to become healthier. They recommend doing moderately intense aerobic exercises. You can spend half an hour every day for five days. But you can do more if you can. The more you exercise, the more fats you burn, so the faster you lose weight.

If you are always running out of time, just make it a point to do any form of exercise, even for as little as ten minutes each day. It can be as simple as going up and down the stairs, biking, or walking to your workplace. If you have kids at home, spend time playing with them. They will love the activity, and you can exercise by doing it. The idea here is always to find ways to be more active.

Focused Thinking about Becoming More Active

Here are some of the thoughts you can add to your list to ensure you will implement changes and be reminded when you forget them:

"I love the energy that being active brings. It makes me happier and joyful to live my life. I love how my body is becoming slimmer. I also love the looks I get from other people and the compliments they say."

"I make sure to walk whenever there's an opportunity to do it. I make it part of my routine. I walk when I need to go somewhere near. I also enjoy walking the dog in the morning and at night."

"I get restless when I haven't exercised yet for the day. It's like my inner voice is nagging me to go out for a while."

"I love the feeling that exercising gives me - the blood flowing easily in my muscles, my heart beating faster, and the urge to move and get something done."

"I always look for opportunities to be active and do something even when I'm busy.

In a Nutshell

This chapter explains why it becomes hard to be active even though it seems too simple to achieve.

- Losing weight is a lifetime commitment and a process.
- Aerobic activity doesn't have to be an exercise. It can be any activity that makes you sweat and breathe harder.
- Lethargy makes you feel stuck when you want to be more active. It's a feeling of not wanting to do anything.
- Lethargy is rooted in many reasons, including lack of self-discipline, attitude and commitment, weakness in character, and more.
- You have to get hold of yourself and control your life before lethargy beats you.
- There are many ways you can do to get past lethargy, including meditation using visualization.
- You also have to develop self-confidence to make it easier to honor your commitments and achieve things.
- Experts suggest adults exercise 150 minutes per week. But you can do more to burn more fat faster.

The next chapter will teach you about reflexology. You can use the knowledge for yourself or administer it to someone you love. It's a form of massage that can help relieve pain, tension, and stress.

CHAPTER TEN

Learning How to Heal Yourself and Others through Reflexology

Weight loss doesn't begin in the gym with a dumbbell; it

starts in your head with a decision.

- Toni Sorenson

Reflexology revolves around the idea that the body can heal itself, which many people tend to ignore. It's an alternative form of healing that is often overlooked due to the presence of medicines and facilities where you can seek treatment no matter your sickness.

Reflexology is a natural healing art that revolves around the idea that the body has reflexes in the hand, face, and feet that match every part of your body. You will need to find these reflexes, stimulate and apply pressure to promote the function and eliminate any aches from which each of your body parts suffers.

Why do you need to learn reflexology?

On your way to a fitter and healthier you, it is only expected to face obstacles along the way, including unexplainable pains. The pains may come from the physical exercises, the sudden change in weather, or your body trying to cope with the changes you keep implementing.

Reflexology helps you deal with the many causes of emotional eating, including stress. It is calming and relaxing. You can learn the process of applying on your own or do it for someone else. You can download reflexology charts for each body part to make it easier to learn the techniques and get it done.

HOW REFLEXOLOGY WORKS

This alternative healing method is best administered by a practitioner who has undergone training about the pressure points in the body. You can do this on your own, with the help of charts and oils to make it easier for you to locate these pressure points. You need to learn how to use your thumbs and hands to stimulate these points and address the body parts to which they correspond.

While reflexology is widely used worldwide to complement other treatment methods for different health problems, it is never intended to cure or diagnose any disorder. It is commonly applied as a preventive measure, especially in health conditions such as anxiety, diabetes, kidney failure, PMS, asthma, and migraines.

Understanding the Reflexology Points and Areas

Some points in the hands, feet, and face correspond to different body organs and parts. It is crucial to locate where these points are and what body parts they correspond to. Even the professionals have used maps of reflex points, which you can download and print or save on your phone.

When you go to a therapist and want to undergo a relaxation session, the reflexologist will work on your ears until your nerves have calmed down. The practice's goal is to release the stress or congestion in your nervous system and give you the right energy balance.

Reflexology is often compared to two other forms of alternative medicine: acupuncture and acupressure. They all work by stimulating the essential points in the body to release the needed energy and try to alleviate the patient's pain. There may be some similarities, but some of the pressure points used in acupuncture and acupressure differ from those used in the reflexology map.

In acupressure, a practitioner traces more than 800 reflex points in the body and are situated along the meridians. The latter is described as thin, long energy lines that run across the body.

Reflexology is also often confused with another form of alternative treatment, massage. Both methods utilize touch but in different approaches. Massage relaxes the muscles through kneading, stroke, tapping, and friction.

Reflexology utilizes what is known as micro-movements. Instead of big and forceful movements like in a massage, a practitioner will walk and hook the reflex points using the thumb or finger until your body responds to the motion. A reflexologist stimulates the nervous system by working from the points found inside your body. Unlike in a full-body massage, you will remain fully clothed during a reflexology session.

Therapeutic Effects of Reflexology

Here are the benefits you can gain from stimulating your reflex areas:

1. Improved vascular and lymphatic circulation

It can boost the blood circulation in your legs, making it helpful to patients with walking or mobility issues. A therapeutic foot massage can lower systolic and diastolic blood pressure and reduce a patient's pulse rate.

2. Neurophysiological benefits

The nervous system benefits the most from the pressure applied to the feet and hands when undergoing reflexology. Studies have shown the relationship between the nervous, endocrine, and immune systems. It normalizes your heart rate and helps you feel more relaxed and happy. It boosts your energy, makes it easier to obtain deep sleep, aids digestion, and relieves stress and anxiety.

3. Balances your energy

The pressure applied to the different points of your body helps you reach the optimum state of homeostasis. The massage unblocks the pathways and balances your energy.

4. Touch

Touch is an effective therapy for people of all ages, no matter what age. Touch is healing and calming. Many nursing homes include touch therapy in how the staff and nurses care for their patients.

A simple touch on the hand or a hug from a loved one has the power to ease the sadness. Touch gives you a feeling that someone cares. It goes through a person's core. It conveys many emotions, such as warmth, love, trust, and respect.

5. Makes you experience ultimate relaxation

The pressure applied to the reflex points in your body relaxes the organs that correspond to them. You will feel relaxed as the blood and energy flow smoothly from within. Your nerves become calm, and you will feel healed by the end of each session.

6. Healing effects

Reflexology helps in relieving migraines and headaches. It eases away your body pains and reduces inflammation. It aids in lowering your blood sugar levels and helps in improving your overall digestive health.

It offers many benefits, many of which target your core. It works on the problems that typically lead to emotional eating.

Reflexology Techniques

To make it easier to self-learn the process, print a reflexology chart you will use as a guide as you follow the techniques. Before learning about the specifics, here are some essential things you need to know about the process. Let us refer to the one getting the massage as the patient. If you administer it to yourself, imagine that you are in the position of the "patient."

1. An ideal session lasts longer than 30 minutes, depending on the age and body built of the patient. If you are attending to an ill patient, an elderly or a young individual, it is not recommended to go beyond 30 minutes.

2. It is not recommended to perform reflexology on people who have been bedridden for more than 24 hours. If they have only recuperated from certain illnesses, their pain tolerance is still low. If they still want the massage, be extra gentle. Frequently pause and ask if they don't get hurt by the pressure.

3. When learning how to perform reflexology, it is recommended to begin with the foot. You will likely find more written studies and research about this type of reflexology since this is widely done in many countries.

4. It is best to do the whole body massage instead of focusing on specific pressure points, depending on the patient's health problems. Perform the whole treatment and spend more time applying pressure to where the pressure points of the patient's health concerns are situated.

5. It is not ideal to use massage oils and creams in performing reflexology. They may help relax and calm the patient's nerves, but they will make it harder for you to exert pressure on your touch, and the skin will be slippery. If you want to use them, apply the oils at the end of the session. Allow their smell and effects to linger on the patient to help them relax after you are done with the massage.

Instead of oils and creams, you can use baby powder when you are performing the massage. The powder will absorb the oils from the patient's body, making it easier for you to apply the needed pressure. Sprinkle the powder on the patient's feet and hands before you begin the process. You can also choose the powder with a pleasant scent that will help your patient relax throughout the massage.

6. The person administering reflexology and the receiver must be comfortable during the session. You can let your patient sit or lie, depending on their preference. If you are

doing the massage, do it at the most comfortable angles. It will reflect on your touch if you are feeling uneasy or awkward. In performing the techniques, it is best not to bend over and never put pressure on your knees.

7. If the patient has diabetes, ask them to check their blood sugar before and after the session. A person may experience a severe rise or drop in blood sugar levels when undergoing this alternative healing.

8. You have to learn the proper techniques you need to use in applying pressure on different body parts. For example, thumb walking is the best technique that can effectively work on the surface of the feet. You can use a circular motion of the index finger in massaging the hands to make the pressure firmer and deeper.

9. People react differently when undergoing a reflexology session. Some will enjoy the process, try to relax, and some fall asleep. Some patients show physical responses during or after the massage. These responses include burping, coughing, spasms, and farting. Some experience tiredness and lack of energy after their first session. You can minimize such reactions by reminding the patient to drink lots of water before and after the session. You must also keep a bottle of water handy during the massage and tell your patient to drink whenever they want to.

FOOT REFLEXOLOGY

You must first learn the thumb walking technique to administer foot reflexology. You can do this for a long time without causing strain to your hand. Let your thumb walk forward by bending and unbending the finger.

Practice your thumbs first and foremost. Look at the upper part of your two thumbs and examine these closely. Roll the top parts of your thumbs until the nails are almost touching. You will use the part where the two thumbs almost touch in the massage.

Use a pen to practice the technique. Hold it with your hand. Use the thumb of your other hand and touch the pen with the part described above. Bend the thumb, allow it to straighten, and repeat the process. As you do this, ensure that the pen does not move, and your thumb stays in contact with it. This is where the pressure will come from

You will exert pressure whenever the thumb is straightened and let the finger move forward as it bends. Start slow. You can do the technique faster as you get the hang of it. You can also practice this on similar surfaces, such as tables and chairs. This technique gives a thorough treatment to the entire foot.

Let's begin.

Always start the session on the right foot. Print out a foot reflexology diagram to make it easier to locate the pressure points in the feet. Here are the steps to get this done:

1. Relax the foot by massaging it all over in a slow manner. Move from the toes to the heel. Do this for 30 seconds or until you feel that the muscles start to relax and loosen up.

Cup the spine area of the foot with the palm of one hand and hold the bottom with the thumb of your other hand. Perform a gentle twist by slowly wringing your hands away from one another. Do this for 30 seconds.

2. Start with the thumb walking action in the spine of the foot. Work from the heel to toes, then down from the toes back to the heel. Do the action from the left to the right direction of the spine until you have covered the entire foot.

3. Hold the big toe and gently rotate it. Do this action to the rest of the toes until you are done with the smallest one. Try to stretch the base joint that holds the toe to the foot as you rotate. This motion works on the bones in your head. This is believed to be effective in relieving headaches.

4. Find the meridian points on the toes, which are situated at the end, except for the middle finger. You will then apply pressure on the meridian point of each toe by making a circular movement. Move the toe clockwise for 10 seconds and counter-clockwise for another 10 seconds. Start with the big toe and work until you are finished with the smallest.

5. Begin the thumb-walk exercise on the toes. Move upwards, following a straight line from the base to the tip. Do this action until you are done with all sides of all toes. The pressure has to be solid and yet, gentle.

Take note that there are certain people whose toes are pretty sensitive. You must first experiment with the pressure and ask them their preference. Never lose the firmness in the pressure. It will tickle your patient if you will perform softly in exerting pressure.

6. You will now perform the massage on the ball of the foot, referred to as the chest region. Do this in a gentle upward motion, downwards, and angular motion until the entire region is covered.

7. Work on the top and back of the foot. Begin from the toes to the ankle and then from the right to the left side of the foot.

8. Look at your printed diagram and see where the waistline is. This is the thinnest part at the bottom part of the foot, and the location may differ from person to person. Thumb walk on the entire area, which corresponds to the liver and stomach.

9. You will now perform the thumb walk between the pelvic region and the waistline.

10. Perform the massage on the pelvic area, which corresponds to the sciatic nerve. Do the action from the left side to the right and then up and at the back of the heel.

11. When you are done, massage the entire foot in a relaxing and gentle manner for a minute.

You are now finished with the right foot. Repeat the steps, but this time, work on the left foot of your patient.

Make sure that you have drinking water on hand during the session. Make the patient drink a big glass of water before you begin. This will help the blood to eliminate the toxins from the body. Advise your patient to keep drinking water the whole day after the session.

FACE REFLEXOLOGY

Face reflexology can be self-administered, but you can also perform this on other people. Before you begin, make sure you have printed out a face reflexology chart so you can locate which areas to work on.

Familiarize yourself with the 15 points in the face. Applying pressure to these points will boost a person's blood circulation, which is a great way to relax. This is typically given to those who want to take a breather and recharge from all the stresses they constantly face.

You can use your index finger or thumb to apply pressure on the reflex points on the face. Push the finger on the pressure point and rotate it without lifting it. Do the action on the same spot, 30 seconds in a clockwise motion and another 30 seconds in the opposite direction.

In performing this kind of reflexology, the patient should be seated. The shoulders and head must be fully supported. Perform the action behind your patient to make it more comfortable for you to move.

1. Stimulate the reflex points in the face one at a time. Follow a diagram and work on the points in sequential order. Work on the whole face before you focus and apply pressure to specific points.

2. Tap the part under the eyes using the tip of the fingers of your two hands. The tapping has to be soft. Tap from the nose to the ears. Rub the jawline with two hands, from the top part of the ears to the chin. Put your index fingers on the chin and begin rubbing for about 15 seconds. Move the fingers from the chin to the edges of the mouth until you reach the cheeks. Circularly rub the cheeks for 30 seconds. Move your fingers to the nose and forehead, and then work on the two eyebrows by rubbing your fingers in an outward motion.

Pull the fingers upwards until you have reached the hairline. Rub this part and then work on the scalp. You can spend as much time as possible in this area because this is extremely relaxing.

3. To maximize the benefits of this reflexology, remind your patient about the importance of water. It has to be taken by the patient before the session and the following hours after. The patient has to take a break and rest after the session.

HAND REFLEXOLOGY

The techniques used in hand reflexology differ from the methods used in giving foot reflexology. The hands are flexible, and the pressure points are deep under the skin. This means that you must exert more effort in pressing and holding the pressure to stimulate the points.

Sit across a table from the patient. Give them a towel that they can place under their hands to offer support. Begin with a relaxation exercise. The hand reflexes are deeper than any of the pressure points in the body. Push the spot using your thumb. Apply a solid but firm pressure. Circularly rotate your thumb for five seconds. Move the thumb to your next target spot and repeat the same steps for another five seconds.

After relaxing the muscles and nerves in the hands, you can begin with hand reflexology by following these steps:

Make sure you first work on the right hand and finish the entire hand before moving to the left one.

1. You can use a bit of baby oil around the wrist of the right hand. Massage the area using a big outward motion with your thumbs. Work your thumbs until you reach the palm of the patient. Massage the inside part of the palm and slowly move towards the edges. Repeat the process for 30 seconds.

Turn the hand over. Using your thumb, begin pushing each knuckle from the bottom to the wrist. Make sure you remain gentle because the action can be painful when too much pressure is applied. Hold a finger at a time. Give each finger a gentle twist from side to side. Gently squeeze the hand to end the relaxation exercise. You can remove the oil by tapping it with a tissue or towel. Perform the same actions on the other hand.

2. Find the meridians in the hands. Circularly work on each meridian, spending five seconds in a clockwise motion and five seconds in a counterclockwise direction. This is how you stimulate the meridians, which include the lung, heart constrictor, colon, heart, small intestine, and the triple burner.

The triple burner meridian does not correspond to any body organ. This pertains to the three major cavities that contain the body organs within. When you stimulate this meridian, you can boost the balance throughout your patient's system.

3. Work on the fingers corresponding to the organs and senses from the neck up. Work from the top part of the thumb of the right hand. Gently move in the direction of the base of the thumb. Cover all thumb areas using the same movement from the top to the base. Work slowly until you have stimulated the whole thumb.

Repeat the process for each of the fingers on the hand you are working on. Work on the part under the little finger. This is beneficial in relieving minor shoulder pains. Pay attention and cover all the skin from the core to the outside areas.

4. Massage the palm corresponding to the body's torso. Lay the hand of the patient on the table with the palm facing upwards. Apply pressure on the soft skin under the fingers, moving downwards and then up and sideways. Do the same procedure to the center of the palm. Spend more time working the base of the thumb and the outer areas of the hand, ensuring that you don't forget any soft padding between the wrist and the palm. This part corresponds to the digestive zone and the spine. Rub the wrist from left to right and repeat, but this time, move in the opposite direction.

5. Turn the hand until the palm is faced down so that you can work on the back of the hand. This part is extra sensitive, so be very gentle in applying pressure. Begin working on the knuckles to the wrist until you are done with all areas. You will then work on the wrist and the wrist bone.

6. Do all the steps mentioned above on the left hand.

You will end the process by doing a round of relaxation exercises for each hand. You can apply a cream or oil this time. Work on the knuckles to the wrist of each hand for 30 seconds. Perform a rubbing motion around the wrist for 15 seconds. Make sure that you cover all areas of the hand. You can add more oil or cream as required. Wring out each finger before you end the exercise for each hand. All your movements need to be slow and gentle. Repeat the process with the other hand.

Hand reflexology is specifically helpful in getting rid of headaches. Like other forms of reflexology, water is essential to make the process effective. Make the patient drink water before the session. Advise them to drink water during the session whenever they feel like it. It is also important that your patient continues to drink more water for the next 24 hours and get sufficient rest.

Other Reminders

Reflexology is a tool that encourages the body to heal on its own. The process is not intended to heal. Instead, it stimulates the different areas and pivotal points in your body to start working and meet their potential to heal. The good thing about the process is that it is safe. It is also quite relaxing and enjoyable.

There are a few cautions that you have to bear in mind to ensure that the process is safe and comfortable for both you and your patient.

Give sufficient water to your patient before, during, and after the session.

If you use scented candles to set the room's ambiance, remember that scented candles can produce too much scent and heat. Use the type with a mild scent and ensure that the room has proper air ventilation.

The massage is best done in a dimly-lit room. It helps in relaxing your patient. If you can't find this space, you can put an eye mask on your patient to achieve the same effect.

In a Nutshell

In this chapter, you've learned a lot about reflexology and how you can use it to relieve yourself from stress and feel better.

- Reflexology is a natural healing art that works around the idea that a human body has reflexes in the hand, face, and feet, which correspond to the different body parts.
- You can do it to yourself but better when you apply it to someone else and let them do the same for you. This way, the pressure will be harder, and it will be easier to locate the reflexes.
- Aside from dealing with the common causes of emotional eating, such as stress and tension, reflexology can help prevent certain sicknesses.
- It is easier if you print or save on your phone a reflexology chart, depending on what you are doing - foot, face, or hand.

CONCLUSION

> *The only bad workout is the one that didn't happen.*
>
> *- Anonymous*

Weight loss is simple. And I still stand to this belief even when we're now at the final part of this piece. It can only be complicated if you make it like that. Once you set your mind to lose weight, you have to stand by it. You can do it one step at a time.

Motivational affirmations help in making things easier to achieve. They give you purpose. They make you believe that you can get things done. They can make you believe in the positive side of things. They imbibe positivity, even when you are feeling down and finding it hard to go on.

Rest your analytical mind when doing affirmations. You can chant or write them, or you can listen to recordings. You can do many affirmations to help you deal with whatever you are facing, such as anxiety affirmations, success affirmations, depression affirmations, and sexual affirmations.

Hypnosis

We have tackled the connection between hypnosis and weight loss. They go hand in hand. It's not enough to deal with the external factors when you deal with weight loss. This will only make you focus on your figure, so you will stop eating, restrict yourself, and take diet pills. You aren't solving the problem this way.

You have to deal with your demons, the inner voice always saying you can't make it, you're depressed, you're ugly, or you are always hungry. You may lose weight this way, but it will only be temporary. You have to get to the roots of the problem, and it is how you feel inside.

You have to tap into your unconscious mind.

You need to understand that you can eat without getting fat, as long as you eat the right amount of the right foods. You have to develop a healthy relationship with food instead of seeing it as an adversary you wouldn't want to get near.

You have to eat only when you are hungry. If your inner voice is still stalling your progress, feed it with positivity by drowning it with affirmations.

To have a healthier relationship with food, you have to meditate while thinking about your future. Imagine yourself as healthy and happy when you reach old age. Make it your goal when you come back to the present time. Always remind yourself that it is what you will become if you succeed in your health goals and plans.

If you have developed emotional eating due to trauma, go back to the day when it started. Visualize the sadness that the trauma brought and the consolation you got from food. Forgive the inner child and tell your young self you're healed, and you no longer need to eat when sad.

Coping with Stress

Stress is among the main culprits why people tend to overeat and binge. It makes you reach for anything so you will get comforted. Stress is not always bad, but it becomes unhealthy when you allow it to have a negative impact on you.

You can do many things to relieve yourself from stress no matter where you are. The techniques depend on the causes. However, the most important steps to deal with stress are talking to others and yourself, taking a break and making stress relief strategies a habit.

Taking Action

To become fit and lose weight fast, you must become more active. You have to take action.

First, you need to know the foods you need to eat to become healthier. Always practice healthy eating. It means you have to supply yourself with the macronutrients in your diet - protein, carbs, or fats. Never restrict your body with these three because it can lead to medical issues and severe malnutrition.

More about Hypnosis

You can follow many hypnosis techniques to help you lose weight, such as reframing, mind disassociation, changing perspectives, and awareness of needs. The gastric band is one of the most effective hypnosis techniques for losing weight. It was patterned after the surgery, but you will only imagine that you had it, how it feels, and what it does to your body, and not undergo the real thing.

Yoga in Promoting Wellbeing

If you haven't been active for a long time and have the urge to exercise more often, it is best to start with activities that only require small movements, such as yoga.

Yoga is a system of exercises and physical poses that can help you become healthier and more fit when done right and regularly. The two most useful aspects of yoga are mudras and asanas. Mudras are hand gestures, and asanas are physical poses. You can also combine the two to gain the most benefits from the process.

What's the Extent of Being Active?

You don't have to perform actual exercises to become active. As long as the movement makes you sweat and your heart beats faster, it is already considered an aerobic activity.

However, there are times when we feel like we're stuck no matter how we put our minds to exercising. You may already be feeling lethargic. It feels like you don't want to do anything. It can be rooted in many factors, including lack of discipline and self-confidence.

You don't have to wait until you lose weight before becoming more confident about yourself. It's a process you need to follow to make it easier for you to have a stronger stance and positive aura.

Learning about Reflexology

When you are on your way to losing weight and keeping your figure, you need all the help you can get. Reflexology is a natural healing art that teaches you how to heal yourself. You can self-administer the massage or do it to your loved one.

Reflexology helps you deal with the various factors that may cause emotional eating. It is healing, calming, and relaxing.

In the end, you will realize that weight loss is a healing journey. Things may not always go as planned, but you will learn something as you go through it. Whenever you feel discouraged, meditate and chant or listen to positive affirmations.

Thank You

You could have picked from dozens of other books, but you picked our book.

Extreme Rapid Weight Loss Hypnosis for Women

So, THANK YOU for getting this book and for making it all the way to the end.

Could you please consider posting a review on Amazon or if you get the Audio version then on Audible?

Posting a positive review is the best and easiest way to support the work of independent authors like me.

Your feedback will help me to keep writing the kind of books that will help you get the results you want.

It can be something short and simple ☺

>> Leave a review on Amazon US <<

>> Leave a review on Amazon UK <<

www.ingramcontent.com/pod-product-compliance
Lightning Source LLC
Chambersburg PA
CBHW070620030426
42337CB00020B/3864